DEDICATION

To all my clients, both past and present. You make this job feel like fun, not work. You inspire me every day with your dedication, your willpower and your awesomeness.

To my long-timers group, those clients who have been with me almost since the beginning — Susan, Vicki, Jane, and Kathi — thanks for trusting me for all these years. I am proud to call myself your friend and it is my honor to work with you.

I0101990

TABLE OF CONTENTS

Introduction

How many diet books have you read in your lifetime? Do you buy the newest book that promises fast and easy weight loss? Do you buy every magazine that announces the latest and greatest new diet on its cover? Are you always looking for the plan that will *finally* help you drop your excess weight and make you feel better in your own skin?

I wish I could tell you that this is *the* book — that finally your magic pill and the perfect plan are within your grasp.

I can't tell you that. But I will tell you that my answers to those questions up above are probably the same as yours. I can also tell you that the majority of diet book authors probably haven't "been there, done that." I have.

Before I became a personal trainer, I was about 30 pounds heavier. Then, as I learned more about health and fitness, and started working out for the first time at the age of 30, I dropped the excess weight and felt great.

Then... a few years ago, I started getting hurt. I teach fitness classes and train clients six days a week. I am constantly lifting and hauling weights around the gym. A few serious injuries forced me to cut way back on strenuous exercise. When I don't exercise frequently enough and intensely enough, I get depressed. When I get depressed, I eat. And when I eat, I don't reach for broccoli...

All of a sudden (well, it was more gradual than sudden, but "gradually" doesn't have the same punch as "all of a sudden") I was 17 pounds heavier than I wanted to be. Great. I developed aches and pains I never had before. My pants were getting tighter in places they shouldn't be tight, and I didn't feel as confident teaching my students and training my clients.

In the past if I gained a few pounds, all I needed to do was exercise a bit more. That didn't work for me now, partly because of my body's limitations with the injuries, and partly because the older we get, the harder it is to lose weight. Lovely, huh?

I would have to focus on my eating.

Ugh.

There was no way I was going on a diet, because all I want to do when I go "on" a diet is go "off" it again. Are you like that? Do you dream of the day you can have a cheeseburger or a cookie or a handful of chips? Do you live for your "cheat" day or meal? Do you go "off" your diet and vow to start again Monday?

Ugh, again.

I don't like living like that. It's not fun. And it doesn't work. At least, not for me.

I finally found something that works for me, and I think it'll work for you.

Before we get into that, you might be wondering who I am, and if I'm qualified to write a diet book.

Well...

My name is Becky Clark. I am not a nutritionist or a doctor. I am not a celebrity or famous athlete, nor do I train celebrities or famous athletes, nor do I look like a celebrity or famous athlete. I don't even *know* any celebrities or famous athletes. And — gasp — I don't have a reality show.

I am just a normal personal fitness trainer (ISSA and NSCA certified, if you care) who works in a normal gym with normal, non-famous people. I've worked with hundreds of clients in the more than ten years I've been a trainer. Normal people. Just like you.

I've spent many, many hours in the gym. I see people there every day who exercise their butts off, yet their bodies don't change much at all, despite their hard work.

Why?

Without speaking to each of these people individually,

my guess is it's their diet. Without a healthy eating plan, all the exercise in the world won't let you lose weight and change your shape. Weight loss is 80% diet (which kind of sucks, if you ask me), and the rest is exercise and genetics.

Trust me on this. As I mentioned earlier, I've struggled with my weight for my entire adult life, especially recently with my injuries. I like to eat. And I hate to diet. I hate to deprive myself of any food (I'm kind of like a tantrum-prone child in that way — the minute you tell me I "can't" have something, I'll throw a tantrum and go have ten of what I "can't" have).

I'd rather eat whatever I want and do extra workouts. But you know what? That doesn't work.

Dammit.

I'll say it again: weight loss is 80% diet.

When I was growing up, eating healthy was as easy as following the four food groups. I wish it was still that simple. I think if it were, we'd have way fewer overweight and obese people in this country, in this world.

There is so much information out there about how to lose weight. One person will tell you the Paleo Diet is the only way to go (lean proteins and veggies, no grains, no processed foods, no beans). Others will tell you a plant-based, vegan diet is healthiest. Others will say to count calories or points. And others will simply say to eat less, move more.

ACK!

It's enough to drive a relatively sane person insane.

It's information overload.

There are some great plans out there, and most of them will help you lose weight. Many of them are healthy. But there's really nothing magical about *any* of them. It all still comes down to cutting calories. Eating less and moving more. Some of these programs just do that in complicated and pretty ways with big words and scientific studies.

Well, you know what? There is no one-size-fits-all diet. Every body is different. You need to find what works for *you* and makes *you* feel good. One of my clients loves eating the Paleo way and feels fabulous. Another tried eating like that and felt bloated with no energy. My doctor is a vegan, with no animal products, and has never looked or felt better. Personally, I like to eat mostly plant-based foods, just because working with and cooking meat makes me kind of sick. (But if someone else makes it, I'm all over it! Yes, I realize I'm weird that way.)

What I'm trying to say is that you need to find a way of eating that you can follow for the rest of your life — because what's the point of losing weight if you're only going to find it again?

Does this sound familiar: When you're "on" a diet, you lose weight. When you're "off" a diet, you gain weight. Yeah. It sucks. It's a vicious cycle, one I am personally familiar with.

But I've usually been able to keep my weight in check because I had a balance between the calories I was feeding my body versus the calories I burned through exercise.

As I said earlier, I hate to diet. That word just makes me cringe and want to binge. I needed to put together a plan I could follow for the rest of my life, without feeling like I was on a diet. Because if I feel like I'm on a diet, I feel like cheating on it. Gee, I'm kind of a brat, aren't I?

I don't usually put together diet plans for my clients (one, because that's not in the scope of my job in the state I live in; and two, because a diet is something people will go off of eventually). What I do is suggest ways they can make their diets a bit healthier according to the goals they've set for themselves. I usually have them start with their worst habit, and go from there.

I needed to do this for myself.

So, I decided to go back to the basics with my eating. I needed something simple and easy to follow. I'm big into lists, so I made a list of my diet "rules" I've shared with my clients over the years. I didn't want to have to follow a "diet" or have to be 100% on my plan. I wanted some wiggle room. If I really want a brownie, I want to be able to have a brownie but not feel like I've failed my eating plan. And not feel like I have to start all over next Monday (after binging all weekend, of course).

Thus, *The Checklist Diet* was born.

Back when I was in school (about a million years ago), I always strove for an A in each class, but I was okay with a B on occasion (and okay, even the occasional C). What if I graded my diet the same way? Strive for an A, be okay with a B, but if I got a C or worse, I needed to work a bit harder. With the checklist, I aimed to follow 10 of 10, but wouldn't beat myself up if I got 9 of 10 (A grade) or even 8 of 10 (B grade). If I got less than that, I still didn't berate myself, I just knew I probably wouldn't see the results I wanted with a C average or worse.

Could it really be this simple? I decided to test it on myself. I'm a 48-year-old, pre-menopausal woman with stubborn lower body fat. Like I said earlier, I'm also like a tantrum-prone child when it comes to following a diet or eating plan. If it's too strict, or it makes me eat something I don't love, I will throw a tantrum — meaning, I will "cheat" on my diet (and once I "cheat", it takes me a while to want to start eating healthy again).

Well, guess what? It *is* that simple. I started this plan on a Monday. Two Mondays later I was down seven pounds with no deprivation, no tantrums, no "cheating" (because there's nothing to "cheat" from). I knew I was on to something.

The steps I'm about to give you are what are working for me, and what work for many of my clients, and what will work for you.

This is not a diet. It's just an easy way to change your eating habits, step by step, and make your diet healthier. I'm not going to spend page after page explaining the science behind weight loss — one, because that's boring, and two, because I don't feel like looking up all that boring stuff. And three, you probably wouldn't read it anyway.

I'm just going to share ten easy steps with you — if you follow most of the steps every day, you will become healthier and leaner than you are now.

Because I am so excited about this diet that is not a diet, I decided to make an affordable e-book for all those people out there just like me who want a healthy, simple way to eat. Who are confused by all the rules. And who, like me, HATE to diet.

The Checklist Diet will work for anyone, unless you're a competitive athlete, a bodybuilder, or a fitness competitor. If you're one of those (and good for you, by the way!), you may need a more structured plan. But for everyone else, all you "normal" people out there just like me, *The Checklist Diet* is the last plan you'll ever need to lose weight and feel great!

Are you ready to learn the easiest way ever to lose weight and follow a healthy diet? Then keep reading!

Author's Note: *As always, please consult with your doctor before making serious changes to your diet. Also, if you have any medical conditions that could be affected by your eating, please talk to your doctor before taking on The Checklist Diet. This book is for educational purposes only. It is not intended to be a substitute for medical advice. Again, I'm neither a nutritionist nor a doctor. "They" told me to tell you all that. I don't know who "they" are, but I tend to listen to them a lot...*

10 Simple Steps to a Better Diet and Healthy Weight Loss

I've come up with 10 simple steps to improve your diet. There is nothing magical or "new" about these steps. You may have heard all this advice before, but maybe you never knew how to put it all together, never understood how to make it your own.

Your goal is to follow at least 8 of the 10 steps every day — that's the ideal. Remember the grading system we talked about earlier? You want to maintain an A or B average.

10 of 10 steps = A+
9 of 10 steps = A
8 of 10 steps = B
7 of 10 steps = C

Less than that...? Don't be mad at yourself or start over on Monday, because there's nothing to start over with. Just try to do better tomorrow. You're always just one meal or snack away from being back on your plan.

So you ate something you shouldn't have, didn't follow the Checklist. So what? No big deal. Just follow the steps the next time you eat.

At the end of each week, review your daily steps, and see if you're skipping the same step or two (or three or four) each day. If so, try really focusing on THAT step for a few days, until it starts to become habit. For me, the step I often fail to follow is #10 — when I've skipped that step more than three days, I take a few days to focus on that. And it never fails to become habit again.

They say it takes 21 days to make a habit. I don't know if that's true — I've never tested the theory and I still don't know "they" — but it sounds good. So I want you to commit to following these 10 steps for 21 days.

If this all still seems overwhelming because your current diet is a total mess (um... been there, done that), maybe you aren't ready for a complete overhaul. I suggest starting with your worst habit. For instance, do you rarely if ever eat breakfast (which is Step #2)? Then start with that step. Once eating a healthy breakfast within an hour of waking up is a habit for you, then move to another step (while continuing with the breakfast habit). Keep adding steps until you're doing all of them most of the time. When you're ready, start aiming for your A or B grade. This is how I did it. I started with my worst habits (Steps 1 & 2), then moved on from there.

Ready for the 10 steps? Okay, here they are. Don't worry — at the end of the book, you'll find them all listed in one place. You can also go to my website and download a copy for yourself. Or, if don't want to deal with flimsy copies, you can order a *Checklist Diet Companion Workbook* (coming soon!), that will let you to track down what you eat and check off the steps all in one convenient place.

Author's Note: Sign up for my newsletter and/or "like" my Facebook page to learn when this book will be available, plus get fitness tips and healthy recipes and learn about my fiction book releases. See the back page of this book for links.

The 10 Steps

Step #1 — Keep track of what you're eating in a food journal or online app.

Ask almost any nutritionist or diet expert what the number one predictor of dieting success is, and they'll tell you it's tracking what you eat. This means either using an online app on your computer or phone (some good ones are Fitday.com and MyFitnessPal.com and LoseIt.com — all free, by the way), or keeping track in a notebook (which is what I did before I created the Checklist Diet Journal). Use whatever is most comfortable and convenient for you.

Several studies have shown that people who keep track of what they're eating are more likely to lose weight and keep it off. In fact, according to "them", dieters who keep a food diary six days a week will lose about twice as much weight as those who track their food one day a week or less. I know that's true for me. If I track my food, and write down EVERYTHING I eat, I will lose weight and/or maintain (depends on my goals); once I stop keeping track, even if I'm choosing healthy foods, I tend to eat more than I should.

You don't necessarily need to track how many calories you're eating or what your macronutrients are (how much protein vs. carbs vs. fats) unless you're into that sort of thing. I'm not. The most important thing is to just write down what you ate. Every single bite. That simple act will hold you accountable. Even though you're the only one who will see this journal, you'll probably refrain from having that second helping of dinner, or nabbing one of your office-mates' doughnuts, because you know you'll have to write it down. Writing down *everything* you eat will also help with mindless munching and emotional eating (two of my biggest problems).

You should, at a minimum, track the time, type, and

amount of food you're eating, and what your hunger level was before you ate. But you don't have to stop there.

You can track more than just the food you're eating. Track your sleep the night before — lack of sleep can prompt us to make poor food choices. There are countless studies out there that will tell you how lack of sleep can affect your weight. (Feel free to Google that — I would do it for you, but I'm kind of busy right now.) People who get the least amount of sleep tend to be the most overweight. That statistic is good enough reason for me to try and get more sleep.

I also like to track my moods throughout the day. I tend to get really tired and grumpy if I've had sugary foods at lunch.

Track how your body feels after a meal. Through tracking my food, I learned that I get sleepy after eating eggs for breakfast. So now if I want eggs, I have them for dinner. Then if they make me tired, I just go to bed. LOL.

At the end of each week, review your food diary. See if you can find any patterns — you can't make a change if you don't know the problem. For example, do you mindlessly reach for food at night before bed even though you're not hungry? Are you constantly skipping certain steps?

If you find some issues, don't beat yourself up about it, just commit to tweaking those problems in the coming week. No biggie.

Step #2 — Eat a healthy, balanced breakfast within an hour of waking up.

When you've been fasting all night, your metabolism and digestion slow down so you can sleep. Think of a car engine that's idling: it's still on, but it's not doing much. When you wake up, you want to fire up that engine as soon as you can in order to start burning more calories—you want to break the fast. The best way to do that is to eat breakfast. Every time you eat, your metabolism speeds up. It's like giving your car some gas, and revving the engine.

Some of my clients don't like to eat breakfast because they say it makes them ravenous later. Well, that's a good thing. That just means your metabolism is revved up, rather than idling. So, rather than waiting until 10 or 11 a.m. to eat your first meal, and have your engine idling and burning fewer calories until that time, why not get a great start to your day by eating breakfast within an hour of waking up?

Notice I said "healthy, balanced breakfast" in Step #2. What does that mean? Come on. You're smart (you picked up this book, didn't you?). You know it doesn't mean a donut and coffee. Or Cap'n Crunch cereal with whole milk. Start with a lean protein (meat, dairy such as yogurt, soy product, or eggs) and add a fruit and/or starchy carb (like cereal or toast). If you love vegetables, breakfast time is a great place for them. *[Check out the food lists at the back of the book.]*

Here are some ideas for healthy breakfasts:
- Whole grain cereal with milk*; half a sliced banana or berries on top
- Oatmeal with skim milk*, a tbsp chopped pecans, 3 chopped frozen cherries
- Whole grain toast with light peanut butter

and an apple
- Scrambled eggs with salsa wrapped inside a whole grain tortilla
- Fruit & protein smoothie (1 cup milk, 1 cup of fruit, 1 scoop protein powder or 6 oz. plain Greek yogurt, squirt of honey)
- Poached egg on toast with just a smidge of butter; ½ cup of berries on the side

When I say "milk", I mean any milk-like product: dairy milk, soy milk, rice milk, almond milk, etc.

If you're really, really, really (I mean really) not hungry when you get up in the morning, and the thought of eating breakfast makes you sick to your stomach, then try having just a few bites of something. Like three slices of apple dipped in peanut butter. Half a piece of toast with light nut butter. A handful of a healthy dry cereal.

After a few days of doing this, the thought of eating a bigger breakfast won't be as unappealing.

Once you're eating a good breakfast every day, it won't take long before you wake up ravenous. Like I said earlier, this is a *good* thing. It means your metabolism is running like a well-oiled engine.

Nice job!

Step #3 — After eating breakfast, eat only when you're hungry.

This is the hardest step for me. I want to eat when I'm bored, when it's "time" to eat, when I'm upset about something. Pretty much any reason other than being hungry. This step is where I differ from many of my fellow trainers. You've probably heard how you *should* eat every 2-3 hours. From a scientific standpoint, this makes sense, because every time you eat, you rev your metabolism. Eating every 2-3 hours give you steady energy, more even-tempered moods (no more low-blood sugar crashes) and could help you to avoid cravings.

But when I eat this way, I'm constantly watching the clock, counting down the minutes until I can eat again, whether I'm hungry or not. Our bodies are very smart. I don't think we need to listen to someone else's rules on when we *should* or *should not* eat. Why don't we just learn to listen to our bodies? When we're hungry, we eat. If we're not hungry, we don't eat. Pretty simple, eh?

Yeah, well "simple" doesn't necessarily mean "easy". Like I said, this is the hardest step for me. But when I follow this step, I automatically drop a few pounds in the first few days.

Some days, you might be hungry all the time. You might eat 5-6 times in a day or even more (but probably not, if you follow all of these 10 steps). But some days, you may only be hungry 2-3 times. OMG, you think. "They" say I need to eat every 3 hours, 5-6x/day!!!!! What to do, what to do????

Calm down and take a deep breath. Like I said, your body is very smart. When you need the fuel (calories) your body will tell you to eat by sending you hunger signals. When you don't need the fuel (maybe you're having a couch potato day), it won't send you many hunger signals, and when you do eat, you'll feel full faster.

Trust me.

Listen to your body.

Most of you will be able to tell when you're hungry and when you're not. Some of you may not like the feeling of being hungry. Well, guess what? If you feel hungry, you get to eat. Isn't that awesome? You don't need to wait for some random time on the clock to eat. No more suffering through hunger pains or a growlingly empty stomach because of the strict diet you're on.

Some of you may not be able to recognize your hunger signals, or don't know what it feels like to be hungry because you've never let yourself get hungry before.

Well, try this: Tomorrow, eat breakfast (Step #1) then check in with your body every 3-4 hours after that. Focus on your stomach. Does it feel empty? Are you getting a bit light-headed or grumpy or spacey? Focus on your mouth. Does it need food?

You're either hungry or you're not. Check in with your body. When your stomach feels empty, it's time to fill it.

If you're not sure if you're hungry or not, you're not.

If you're thinking you SHOULD be hungry because you haven't eaten in a while, or you SHOULD be hungry because this is the time of day you usually eat, then you're not listening to your body.

Think of your hunger as a scale of 1-10.
    10 — Thanksgiving stuffed
    7 — You feel like you ate a bit too much and are
        slightly uncomfortable
    5 — Comfortable
    3 — You're a little bit hungry, but you could wait
    0 — Your stomach is empty and you need to eat

"But I'm *always* hungry," you might say. Maybe, maybe not. It's probably head hunger (you are craving something or want to eat for emotional reasons). But maybe you ARE always hungry. That's okay. That's your body's way of telling you it needs fuel. Make sure you're eating enough (see Step #10) and your body will regulate itself. (*Remember, if you're a competitive athlete, or are training for some sort of competition, this way of eating may not work for you. For us normal people, this way of eating will work just fine.)

Author's note: If emotional eating is a problem for you, check out any book by Geneen Roth, or the book *Intuitive Eating* by Evelyn Tribole & Elyse Resch. If you think emotional eating is a *big* problem for you, please consider speaking to a professional.

Step #4 — Combine a protein and a "good" carb every time you eat.

You'll want to eat a lean protein every time you eat, because this will help fuel your body efficiently, support muscle growth, boost your metabolism, keep your energy levels on an even keel, and keep those cravings at bay.

What is a protein? Here are some examples (also check out the food lists at the back of the book):

- Eggs
- Lean meat (beef, chicken, turkey, pork)
- Fish
- Cottage cheese
- Yogurt
- Beans
- Nuts & Seeds
- Quinoa (a grain that's also a complete protein)
- Nut butter
- Tofu or other soy products

My views on protein are another area where many of my peers and I differ. Many of them insist protein means *animal* protein, such as lean meats, eggs, dairy products. I'm not saying you can't eat those foods. If you enjoy them, go for it. But if you are more like me and don't enjoy eating so much animal protein, then you don't have to. It's no big deal. As I said before, there is no one-size-fits-all diet out there, no matter what the "experts" want to tell you. With this plan, you can choose the types of protein that *you* like to eat. Period. (See the food lists at the back of the book for more ideas.)

Now, let's talk about carbohydrates. No, that's not a four-letter word (well, "carb" is a four-letter word, but you won't get in trouble here for saying it out loud). Yes, you can eat carbs. No, carbs are not the enemy. Yes, I know Dr. Atkins, the Paleo diet people, and others have drilled into your head over and over for years that carbs make you fat. Well, they don't. Unless you overeat them. And unless you eat the wrong kinds of carbs — like donuts, white bread, foods with white flour, sugary cereals, etc.

First of all, let's be clear what constitutes a carbohydrate.

All fruits and vegetables are carbohydrates.

Breads, pastas, rice, oatmeal, potatoes are carbs.

Legumes, quinoa, rye berries, millet are carbs.

Donuts, foods made with white flour, sugary cereal, etc. are also carbs, but you're smart. You know you shouldn't be eating them. At least not very often. But when in doubt, choose from the food lists at the back of the book.

Everything in moderation, people.

Over the years, I've tried pretty much all of the popular diets, because I knew at least one of my clients would probably try it. By learning about the program and trying it for myself (unless it sounded dangerous and/or stupid), I could discuss it rationally with my clients. So, yes, I've tried the no-carb/low-carb thing. And you know what? I lost weight. You know what else? I hated every minute of it. I felt bloated and had no energy to sustain my workouts and crazy work schedule. You know what else? I gained back the weight I lost and then some, because it wasn't a diet I could sustain. But I have a friend who eats the Paleo way and does Crossfit (crazy intense workouts) and she feels great.

Maybe *you're* happy eating a lot of meat and few/no starchy carbs. Maybe this way of eating makes you feel great. Well, that's awesome. Some of my clients feel the exact same way. But you still need carbohydrates in the way of vegetables and fruits. *Lots* of vegetables and fruits (we'll talk more about them in Step #5).

So I'll say it again: LISTEN TO YOUR BODY. Eat the way that feels best for you.

Why do you need carbohydrates? For energy, pure and simple. Some of us need more than others. It depends on your body type and energy expenditure. It's been my experience with my clients (and now I've read studies that back up my observations) that those people who have "apple" shapes — you carry your extra weight in your torso — are often carbohydrate sensitive. You can still eat starchy carbs, but try limiting them to 1-2 servings a day, and not eating them after the noon hour. People who are "pear" shaped, like me — you carry your extra weight in your hips, thighs and butt — don't have a problem eating starchy carbs as long as you don't overeat them.

Here is a good rule of thumb: when eating a starchy carb (see food list at the end of the book), keep your portion size no bigger than the size of your closed fist. And eat only one starchy carb per meal/snack (1-2x/day if you're apple shaped). If you do those two things, it'll be virtually impossible to overeat your starchy carbs.

If your starchy carb comes in a package (like rice or pasta or bread), you can also read the serving size on the label to figure out what *one* portion is.

This rule might sound complicated, but it's not. A snack could be as simple as celery or apple with nut butter. Yogurt and berries. A hardboiled egg and a piece of fruit. Half of a tuna salad sandwich on whole grain bread. The possibilities are endless.

Step #5 —Eat a fruit or vegetable every time you eat. Aim for 5 total servings — 2 fruits and 3+ veggies a day.

Our moms and grandmas always told us to eat our veggies, and they were right! The quickest and easiest way to improve your diet and to lose weight is to eat more produce and less junk food. When you're hungry, reach for a piece of fruit instead of a candy bar. You'll still get the sweetness you crave but for a fraction of the calories.

Fruits and vegetables are chock full of vitamins, minerals, and fiber that you just can't get in a pill or any other food. They'll fill you up, they'll improve the look of your skin, and they'll give you tons of energy. My goal is always to make half of my daily food intake produce. Do I always meet that goal? Oh, hell no. But when I do, my energy is boundless and my skin looks great!

Why am I limiting you to just two fruits a day? Isn't fruit good for you? Yes, it's really good for you. I'm pretty sure nobody ever got fat from eating too much fruit. However, fruit is sweet because it's full of sugar. And too much sugar of any kind can pack on the calories and the pounds.

Now, here's a slight caveat for you: If you're apple shaped, meaning you carry your excess weight in your torso, then stick to the 2 servings a day, because your body type may not be able to metabolize carbohydrates well. You could even try replacing those two servings with extra veggies for quicker results. But if you carry your weight in the lower body, you could have three servings a day. If you carry your extra weight evenly throughout your body, I'd stick with two servings until you're at your goal weight.

I have to be honest with you... I don't love veggies. In fact, I don't really even LIKE most of them. I force myself to have a big salad several times a week, because raw vegetables are more appealing to me. But the easiest way I've found to get my fruit and vegetable servings in is by making a smoothie most days.

Here's my favorite (warning: it looks like something out of the Exorcist):

The It-Tastes-Better-Than-It-Looks Smoothie

- ½ cup frozen fruit (I like a mix of strawberries and cherries; this works out to about 2 whole strawberries and 3 cherries)
- 1 cup almond milk (or other skim milk of choice)
- 1 tbsp ground flaxseed
- 2 tsp nut butter (my fave is almond butter)
- Drizzle of honey or Agave or Xylitol
- *Ice is optional — add some if you like a thicker smoothie
- 1 scoop protein powder of choice (I use brown rice protein powder — it's an acquired taste and is actually pretty disgusting the first time you try it. Vanilla or chocolate whey powder would also work.)
- Fill the rest of the blender with raw spinach

Blend until everything is mixed. It will be an ugly brownish green color, but you won't taste the spinach, I promise.

Step #6 — Eat 25 grams of fiber each day.

Growing up, I always heard about how I should eat more fiber. That I'd lose weight if I ate enough fiber. That fiber keeps you "regular" and that it's good for your health. All those statements are true. But somewhere along the way, over the past few years, people stopped talking about fiber — maybe because it's not sexy like "high protein" and "low carb" and "gluten-free."

But here's the thing. You need fiber. Why? Because numerous studies have shown that getting enough fiber lowers your risk for coronary heart disease, obesity, and certain cancers. Fiber also will make you feel full faster, which could help you eat less. Pretty cool, eh?

Unfortunately, you're probably not getting enough.

According to WebMD, the average person takes in about 15 g of fiber a day, but most experts say women need 25 g and men need 38 g. It's really not that hard if you're eating a lot of fruits, vegetables, and whole grains. If you're on the Paleo or low-carb bandwagon, you *might* not be getting enough.

Look how quickly your fiber intake could stack up:

- pear with skin: 5.5 g
- apple with skin: 5 g
- 1 c. raspberries: 8 g
- 1 c. whole wheat spaghetti: 6.3 g
- 1 c. pearl barley: 6 g
- 1 c. cooked lentils: 15.6 g
- 1 c. cooked black beans: 15 g
- 1 oz. raw almonds: 3.5 g
- 1 medium artichoke: 10.3 g
- 1 c. broccoli: 5.1 g

Check out the food lists in the back for more options.

If you have a high-fiber food with every snack or meal, you'll easily meet your fiber quota. But here's a word of warning — if you haven't been eating much fiber, please build up your intake slowly. Otherwise, your tummy will be yelling at you. Then you'll be yelling at me. And that'll make me very sad.

One more thing — be sure to drink enough water when you increase your fiber intake. See Step #7 for more on water.

Step #7 — Drink 8-10 glasses of water daily.

You've probably heard this recommendation before, but maybe you're not sure why it's so important to drink your water. Well, I'll tell you. Our bodies are about 60% water, our brains are 75% water by weight, and muscle is about 80% water. It follows, then, that if we're not hydrating enough and sufficiently, our entire body will suffer. All the systems in your body will function better if you're well hydrated.

Don't rely on your thirst signals to drink water, because once you actually feel thirsty, you're probably already dehydrated. Look at the color of your urine. If it's dark yellow, you're dehydrated. If it's light in color, you're doing pretty well. Everyone's dehydrated in the morning, so you should try to get into the habit of drinking a tall glass of plain water first thing when you wake up each morning.

We lose fluids constantly just going about our day-to-day lives — through skin evaporation, urine, sweating (from warm temps and from exercise), high altitudes, etc. If your fluid input doesn't equal your output, you'll become dehydrated.

Water also helps you lose weight by controlling calories. There's nothing magical about this: if you drink plain water instead of a beverage containing calories, you'll save those calories. And every little bit helps. For example, if you substitute plain water (0 calories) for just one can of regular soda (approx. 140 calories) every day, you'll save 51,100 calories a year, and could lose more than 14 pounds from that change alone. (It generally takes a loss of 3500 calories to lose a pound.)

Signs of mild to moderate dehydration:

- Dry mouth

- Thirst
- Sleepiness/tiredness
- Dark yellow or gold urine (all of us are dehydrated in the morning, so drink a cup of water first thing when you wake up)
- Dry skin
- Constipation
- Headache (when I get a headache, I immediately pound a tall glass of water. That usually takes care of it.)
- Dizziness or lightheadedness

This should be the easiest of all these steps to accomplish. I mean, everyone likes water, right?

Wrong.

I really don't like water. The only time I enjoy it is in the middle of a workout. Because I don't enjoy it, I rarely think of drinking it. So I need to give myself reminders.

Easy ways to get more water into your diet:

- I keep bottled water in the trunk of my car, and have an open one in my beverage holder at all times (room temp water goes down easier for me).
- I bought one of those cool 32 oz. reusable cups with straws from Starbucks. In fact, I have about 5 or 6 of them floating around my house. I keep one of them on the counter, filled with water. Once I started doing that, I was really proud of how much water I was drinking. And it seemed effortless. Turns out, it *was* effortless — my daughter had been drinking out of the cup, too. She was the one drinking all the water. LOL. Well, at least one of us was hydrated.
- Eat more fruits and vegetables. (See Step

#5.) The more water-based foods you eat, the less actual water you have to drink.

- Have a cup of green or herbal tea every afternoon instead of a coffee break.
- Eat a bowl of soup for lunch and/or dinner (high in water content).
- One of my clients puts 6 bracelets on her left arm every morning, each one representing a glass of water. Her goal is to get them all to her right arm by the time she goes to bed each night.
- Another client puts 4 rubber bands around his 16 oz. water bottle each morning. Every time he empties the bottle, he takes off a rubber band.
- Drink an 8 oz. glass every time you eat.

Step #8 — Stop eating 2 hours before bedtime.

You've probably heard this rule before, too. There's nothing magical about it. Digestion takes a lot of energy. If you eat too close to bedtime, you'll expend so much energy digesting your food, you may have trouble sleeping and getting the rest you need.

But the main reason I put this down as a step is because the night time, after dinner, is many people's weak time. We're getting tired, and our willpower sometimes gets tired too. Now, if we're reaching for broccoli or brown rice when our willpower sags, that wouldn't be so bad. But most of us pick foods like popcorn, ice cream, chips, candy. It's been a long day, we're tired, we just want to sit in front of the TV and munch. A handful (or more) of chips would taste so good. Or some buttered popcorn. Or another serving from dinner. But by following this step, you'll eliminate this problem.

It's okay to go to bed a little bit hungry. I'll repeat that last part: a *little bit* hungry. But if you're absolutely starving and it's less than 2 hours until bedtime, you need to eat. Maybe you get home from work or the gym at 8 and need to be in bed by 10. You don't need to refrain from eating if that's your situation. If you're really hungry, please eat. Just make a healthy choice, okay? And make it a small serving. But the rest of you? Just say no.

Step #9 — No Junk Food & Limit Your Alcohol.

If you think it might be bad for you, it probably is.

This one is kind of a no-brainer, isn't it? I can tell just by looking at you that you're pretty smart. You know instinctively what food is "good" for you and what food is "bad" for you. Come on — you know that a Big Mac and fries are not good for you. You know that a candy bar or a bag of potato chips is not good for you.

Am I saying you can never have these things? No. You can actually have some sort of junk food every day — I didn't say you had to have 100% compliance with this checklist. If you get 8 of 10 items checked every day, that leaves a little wiggle room. There are some days I absolutely MUST eat a candy bar. Some times I want one every day for a few days. Well then, I just make sure I'm following ALL of the other steps that day. Sometimes, just telling myself that I could have some chocolate if I really wanted some is enough. It's like I'm a toddler having a tantrum. "I want some! I don't care if you said I can't. I want some!" Well, once I tell my inner toddler that I can have some chocolate/chips/whatever if I really want it, I usually don't really want it after all.

Now, let's talk alcohol consumption. Don't freak out. I'm not telling you that you can't drink. I'm just telling you to not drink *too much*. And here's why. One, it's full of empty calories. Alcohol contains 7 calories per gram and offers no nutritional value. It only adds empty calories to your diet. Wouldn't you rather spend your calories on healthier fare? Two, drinking may lower your inhibitions as far as eating right goes — with a couple of beers or glasses of wine in you, you may be more inclined to overeat, or eat something you "shouldn't." In fact, alcohol has been proven to stimulate the appetite. Yikes. I don't need *anything* to stimulate my appetite. I do this quite nicely on my own, thank you very much. Three, it'll fill you up, which will curb your hunger. And when you're hungry, you should really be filling your gut with nutritious foods, not with empty calories like alcohol.

Your body also doesn't metabolize alcohol very well. According to WebMD, alcohol consumption is associated with bigger waists. Each drink you have contains calories. And the food you eat with that drink has calories, too.

If you drink too much, guess where it'll go? Have you ever seen a guy who drinks too much beer? Have you seen his beer belly? It's called that for a reason. According to a recent Swiss study, when you drink alcohol, your body burns fat more slowly than usual. Alcohol throws off the body's normal disposal of fat in the diet.

And fat that is not burned is stored in your gut, your thighs, or wherever else you tend to store fat. Like your butt.

Oh. My. God. Not only could you get a beer belly, you could get a beer *butt*.

Yikes.

"But Becky," you say, "I've heard that having a drink every day is good for me." I've heard that, too. Many experts say that consuming a *single* drink per day can have certain health benefits. However, if you're having more than one drink daily, you could be sabotaging your health and weight loss goals.

Step #10 — Stop eating when satisfied, not full.

This one tip might be the most important for you in terms of weight loss. And this step is the absolutely most difficult one for me.

Most of us eat beyond satisfied. Most of us eat until full or beyond. And if you are in the habit of eating until full or beyond, you probably won't lose weight, no matter what kind of food you are eating. (Okay, if you're stuffing yourself silly on raw celery, you might be okay. But then I'd have to question your sanity... so you might *not* be okay...)

Your stomach can only handle so much food at once. Think about this: your stomach is about the size of your closed fist. And unfortunately, it's very flexible. Which means it'll stretch to accommodate a feast. But honestly — when was the last time you ate just a fist-sized amount of food?

Like I said earlier, this is the hardest step for me, especially if I'm eating something really, really yummy.

Speaking of really, really yummy... *Hara hachi bu.* No, I didn't just sneeze. It's a Japanese saying that means, "Eat until you're 80% full." The Okinawans, who are known for their health and longevity, follow this cultural habit of calorie control. Which is probably why they have much less incidence of obesity in their society than we do. We eat too much, plain and simple.

Another trick to help you stop overeating is the Three-Bite Rule. This means stop eating when the food stops tasting so good, which is usually after about three bites. Think about the last time you had a fabulous dessert. Those first couple of bites were amazing. But after that, that awesomeness faded to just pretty good. If you could get into the habit of eating until the point where it downgrades from amazing, your waistline would thank you.

I don't follow this particular suggestion for every food I eat, because there are few foods I find "amazing." If I followed this rule when eating vegetables or some of my other healthy cooking, I'd never eat. LOL. However, when eating dessert or candy or something else "bad" I've been craving, I usually follow this tip. And you know what? It's really true. After those first couple of bites, which I savor and really enjoy, I don't really want more.

Try it. You'll see.

Next time you have the craving for something amazing and sinful (like cheesecake), take the first bite and savor the deliciousness. Eat it slowly. Now, take another bite. It probably tastes almost as good, although the first bite is always the best. Take a third bite. Doesn't taste any better, does it? Now, take a fourth bite. Does it still taste as fabulous as the first couple of bites? Probably not. If not, why would you keep eating it? Your taste buds are telling you to stop. Stop after three delicious and guilt-free bites and you'll never overeat a dessert or treat again.

Back to Step #10. If you get into the habit of eating just until your stomach is full (to its capacity without stretching), you'll lose weight.

Remember the hunger scale we talked about in Step #3?

If you consistently eat in the range of 0 to 5 on the hunger scale, you'll lose weight.

If you consistently eat in the range of 3 to 7 on the hunger scale, you'll stay at the weight you are now.

If you consistently eat in the range of 5 to 10 on the hunger scale, you'll gain weight.

Did you see the key word up there? "Consistently"?

Eating until over full on occasion won't hurt you, but *consistently* eating this way will cause you to gain weight.

Simply wait until your stomach is empty before filling it again. If you do this, you'll lose weight. You almost can't help it.

Putting it all together

There you have it. Those are the not-so-magic steps. I told you it was simple.

"Wait a doggone minute, Becky!" you say. "Where is the cheat day?"

There's no need for "cheat days" or "cheat meals" on this plan, because they're built into the Checklist. Remember, you're aiming for an A or B grade (8-10 items checked) every day.

If you really want a brownie (which would be not following Step #9), then have a brownie, but make sure you follow all the other steps. See? No need for a cheat day or cheat meal with this plan.

For instance, yesterday I really, really, really wanted a cheeseburger. So I had one for lunch. And I really, really, really enjoyed it. I just made sure I followed all the other steps. I waited until I was hungry (Step #3) to eat that cheeseburger, and I ordered some sliced apples to go with it (Step #5), and I stopped eating when I was satisfied, not full (Step #10), which was easy because it was a small burger and it didn't fill me up, so I was able to eat the whole thing without a lick of guilt. And you know what? It was awesome. Now, for the rest of the week, I'll try not to skip that step of avoiding junk food (Step #9). But if I really want a brownie tomorrow, I'll make it work.

Remember to review your daily checklists at the end of each week. Are you skipping the same steps every day? For instance, are you consistently NOT checking off Step #2 (eat breakfast) and Step #6 (eat enough fiber)? Then those are the steps you probably need to work on for a while.

How will you know if this plan is working for you?

Well, are you losing weight (if that's your goal) and feeling great? Then it's working for you. Keep doing what you're doing. And you might find that you can be successful by only being 70% compliant. Or even 60%. It depends what "successful" means to you. It depends what steps you're consistently following or not following. For instance, if I need to drop a few pounds (like after Thanksgiving) and I consistently follow Steps 1, 2 and 10, I will lose weight whether or not I'm following the other steps. But it's not just about weight loss for me. It's about eating a healthy diet, so I still strive for an A or B grade.

If you're just wanting to improve your diet a bit and you don't really care about weight loss, just adding a few of these steps into your daily routine might be all you need. But if you want 100% success, you must have 100% compliance.

Do I have 100% compliance 100% of the time? Oh, hell no. Life's too short to not have the occasional Big Mac or Girl Scout cookie. But... I am honest with myself. If I am 70% consistent or less, I will probably gain weight, and definitely won't have the energy I need to get through my busy days. I need 80% consistency or better. I know that because I've done less. I've tested this system.

These are the steps that work for me. They work for many of my clients. They'll work for you, too.

THE DAILY CHECKLIST
Day & Date _____

☐ 1. Keep track of what you're eating

☐ 2. Eat breakfast within an hour of waking up.

☐ 3. Wait until you are hungry to eat (except for rule #2).

☐ 4. Eat protein & carb at every meal/snack.

☐ 5. Eat a vegetable or fruit every time you eat.

    Fruit ☐ ☐ | Vegetables ☐ ☐ ☐

☐ 6. Eat 25 g of fiber each day. Today approx. total: _____ g

☐ 7. Drink 8-10 glasses of water daily. ☐ ☐ ☐ ☐ ☐ ☐ ☐ ☐ ☐

☐ 8. Stop eating 2 hours before bedtime.

☐ 9. No junk food & limited alcohol.

☐ 10. Stop eating when satisfied, not full.

How many steps did you follow today? ___/10

What was your "grade" today? __ (A or B is your goal)

9 or 10/10 = A
8 of 10 = B
7 of 10 = C
Less than that? Just strive for better tomorrow, okay? No big deal. Remember, you're always just one meal or snack away from being back on your plan.

How was your energy level today?

How were your moods today?

How many hours did you sleep last night?

What step (if any) do you need to focus on tomorrow?

Daily Food Diary

Hunger Scale:

10   Thanksgiving stuffed--You ate too much and are slightly uncomfortable

5   Comfortable

3   You're a little bit hungry, but you could wait

0   Your stomach is empty

Try to eat in the range of 0 to 5 for best results

TIME	FOOD	Hunger # before eating	Hunger # after eating

THE DAILY CHECKLIST

Day & Date _____

☐ 1. Keep track of what you're eating

☐ 2. Eat breakfast within an hour of waking up.

☐ 3. Wait until you are hungry to eat (except for rule #2).

☐ 4. Eat protein & carb at every meal/snack.

☐ 5. Eat a vegetable or fruit every time you eat.

    Fruit ☐ ☐ | Vegetables ☐ ☐ ☐

☐ 6. Eat 25 g of fiber each day. Today approx. total: _____ g

☐ 7. Drink 8-10 glasses of water daily. ☐ ☐ ☐ ☐ ☐ ☐ ☐ ☐ ☐

☐ 8. Stop eating 2 hours before bedtime.

☐ 9. No junk food & limited alcohol.

☐ 10. Stop eating when satisfied, not full.

How many steps did you follow today? __/10

What was your "grade" today? __ (A or B is your goal)

9 or 10/10 = A
8 of 10 = B
7 of 10 = C
Less than that? Just strive for better tomorrow, okay? No big deal. Remember, you're always just one meal or snack away from being back on your plan.

How was your energy level today?

How were your moods today?

How many hours did you sleep last night?

What step (if any) do you need to focus on tomorrow?

Daily Food Diary

Hunger Scale:

10	Thanksgiving stuffed--You ate too much and are slightly uncomfortable
5	Comfortable
3	You're a little bit hungry, but you could wait
0	Your stomach is empty

Try to eat in the range of 0 to 5 for best results

TIME	FOOD	Hunger # before eating	Hunger # after eating

THE DAILY CHECKLIST

Day & Date _____

☐ 1. Keep track of what you're eating

☐ 2. Eat breakfast within an hour of waking up.

☐ 3. Wait until you are hungry to eat (except for rule #2).

☐ 4. Eat protein & carb at every meal/snack.

☐ 5. Eat a vegetable or fruit every time you eat.

    Fruit ☐ ☐ | Vegetables ☐ ☐ ☐

☐ 6. Eat 25 g of fiber each day. Today approx. total: _____ g

☐ 7. Drink 8-10 glasses of water daily. ☐ ☐ ☐ ☐ ☐ ☐ ☐ ☐ ☐

☐ 8. Stop eating 2 hours before bedtime.

☐ 9. No junk food & limited alcohol.

☐ 10. Stop eating when satisfied, not full.

How many steps did you follow today? __/10

What was your "grade" today? __ (A or B is your goal)

9 or 10/10 = A
8 of 10 = B
7 of 10 = C
Less than that? Just strive for better tomorrow, okay? No big deal. Remember, you're always just one meal or snack away from being back on your plan.

How was your energy level today?

How were your moods today?

How many hours did you sleep last night?

What step (if any) do you need to focus on tomorrow?

Daily Food Diary

Hunger Scale:

10   Thanksgiving stuffed--You ate too much and are slightly uncomfortable

5   Comfortable

3   You're a little bit hungry, but you could wait

0   Your stomach is empty

Try to eat in the range of 0 to 5 for best results

TIME	FOOD	Hunger # before eating	Hunger # after eating

THE DAILY CHECKLIST

Day & Date _____

☐ 1. Keep track of what you're eating

☐ 2. Eat breakfast within an hour of waking up.

☐ 3. Wait until you are hungry to eat (except for rule #2).

☐ 4. Eat protein & carb at every meal/snack.

☐ 5. Eat a vegetable or fruit every time you eat.

    Fruit ☐ ☐ | Vegetables ☐ ☐ ☐

☐ 6. Eat 25 g of fiber each day. Today approx. total: _____ g

☐ 7. Drink 8-10 glasses of water daily. ☐ ☐ ☐ ☐ ☐ ☐ ☐ ☐ ☐

☐ 8. Stop eating 2 hours before bedtime.

☐ 9. No junk food & limited alcohol.

☐ 10. Stop eating when satisfied, not full.

How many steps did you follow today? ___/10

What was your "grade" today? __ (A or B is your goal)

9 or 10/10 = A
8 of 10 = B
7 of 10 = C
Less than that? Just strive for better tomorrow, okay? No big deal.
Remember, you're always just one meal or snack away from being
back on your plan.

How was your energy level today?

How were your moods today?

How many hours did you sleep last night?

What step (if any) do you need to focus on tomorrow?

Daily Food Diary

Hunger Scale:

10   Thanksgiving stuffed--You ate too much and are slightly uncomfortable

5   Comfortable

3   You're a little bit hungry, but you could wait

0   Your stomach is empty

Try to eat in the range of 0 to 5 for best results

TIME	FOOD	Hunger # before eating	Hunger # after eating

THE DAILY CHECKLIST
Day & Date _____

☐ 1. Keep track of what you're eating

☐ 2. Eat breakfast within an hour of waking up.

☐ 3. Wait until you are hungry to eat (except for rule #2).

☐ 4. Eat protein & carb at every meal/snack.

☐ 5. Eat a vegetable or fruit every time you eat.

    Fruit ☐ ☐ | Vegetables ☐ ☐ ☐

☐ 6. Eat 25 g of fiber each day. Today approx. total: _____ g

☐ 7. Drink 8-10 glasses of water daily. ☐ ☐ ☐ ☐ ☐ ☐ ☐ ☐ ☐

☐ 8. Stop eating 2 hours before bedtime.

☐ 9. No junk food & limited alcohol.

☐ 10. Stop eating when satisfied, not full.

How many steps did you follow today? ___/10

What was your "grade" today? __ (A or B is your goal)

9 or 10/10 = A
8 of 10 = B
7 of 10 = C
Less than that? Just strive for better tomorrow, okay? No big deal. Remember, you're always just one meal or snack away from being back on your plan.

How was your energy level today?

How were your moods today?

How many hours did you sleep last night?

What step (if any) do you need to focus on tomorrow?

Daily Food Diary

Hunger Scale:

10   Thanksgiving stuffed--You ate too much and are slightly uncomfortable

5   Comfortable

3   You're a little bit hungry, but you could wait

0   Your stomach is empty

Try to eat in the range of 0 to 5 for best results

TIME	FOOD	Hunger # before eating	Hunger # after eating

THE DAILY CHECKLIST

Day & Date _____

☐ 1. Keep track of what you're eating

☐ 2. Eat breakfast within an hour of waking up.

☐ 3. Wait until you are hungry to eat (except for rule #2).

☐ 4. Eat protein & carb at every meal/snack.

☐ 5. Eat a vegetable or fruit every time you eat.

   Fruit ☐ ☐ | Vegetables ☐ ☐ ☐

☐ 6. Eat 25 g of fiber each day. Today approx. total: _____ g

☐ 7. Drink 8-10 glasses of water daily. ☐ ☐ ☐ ☐ ☐ ☐ ☐ ☐ ☐

☐ 8. Stop eating 2 hours before bedtime.

☐ 9. No junk food & limited alcohol.

☐ 10. Stop eating when satisfied, not full.

How many steps did you follow today? ___/10

What was your "grade" today? __ (A or B is your goal)

9 or 10/10 = A
8 of 10 = B
7 of 10 = C
Less than that? Just strive for better tomorrow, okay? No big deal.
Remember, you're always just one meal or snack away from being
back on your plan.

How was your energy level today?

How were your moods today?

How many hours did you sleep last night?

What step (if any) do you need to focus on tomorrow?

Daily Food Diary

Hunger Scale:

10   Thanksgiving stuffed--You ate too much and are slightly uncomfortable

5   Comfortable

3   You're a little bit hungry, but you could wait

0   Your stomach is empty

Try to eat in the range of 0 to 5 for best results

TIME	FOOD	Hunger # before eating	Hunger # after eating

THE DAILY CHECKLIST

Day & Date _____

☐ 1. Keep track of what you're eating

☐ 2. Eat breakfast within an hour of waking up.

☐ 3. Wait until you are hungry to eat (except for rule #2).

☐ 4. Eat protein & carb at every meal/snack.

☐ 5. Eat a vegetable or fruit every time you eat.

　　　Fruit ☐ ☐ | Vegetables ☐ ☐ ☐

☐ 6. Eat 25 g of fiber each day. Today approx. total: _____ g

☐ 7. Drink 8-10 glasses of water daily. ☐ ☐ ☐ ☐ ☐ ☐ ☐ ☐ ☐

☐ 8. Stop eating 2 hours before bedtime.

☐ 9. No junk food & limited alcohol.

☐ 10. Stop eating when satisfied, not full.

How many steps did you follow today? ___/10

What was your "grade" today? __ (A or B is your goal)

9 or 10/10 = A
8 of 10 = B
7 of 10 = C
Less than that? Just strive for better tomorrow, okay? No big deal.
Remember, you're always just one meal or snack away from being
back on your plan.

How was your energy level today?

How were your moods today?

How many hours did you sleep last night?

What step (if any) do you need to focus on tomorrow?

Daily Food Diary

Hunger Scale:

10   Thanksgiving stuffed--You ate too much and are slightly uncomfortable

5   Comfortable

3   You're a little bit hungry, but you could wait

0   Your stomach is empty

Try to eat in the range of 0 to 5 for best results

TIME	FOOD	Hunger # before eating	Hunger # after eating

THE DAILY CHECKLIST

Day & Date _____

☐ 1. Keep track of what you're eating

☐ 2. Eat breakfast within an hour of waking up.

☐ 3. Wait until you are hungry to eat (except for rule #2).

☐ 4. Eat protein & carb at every meal/snack.

☐ 5. Eat a vegetable or fruit every time you eat.

   Fruit ☐ ☐ | Vegetables ☐ ☐ ☐

☐ 6. Eat 25 g of fiber each day. Today approx. total: _____ g

☐ 7. Drink 8-10 glasses of water daily. ☐ ☐ ☐ ☐ ☐ ☐ ☐ ☐ ☐

☐ 8. Stop eating 2 hours before bedtime.

☐ 9. No junk food & limited alcohol.

☐ 10. Stop eating when satisfied, not full.

How many steps did you follow today? ___/10

What was your "grade" today? __ (A or B is your goal)

9 or 10/10 = A
8 of 10 = B
7 of 10 = C
Less than that? Just strive for better tomorrow, okay? No big deal. Remember, you're always just one meal or snack away from being back on your plan.

How was your energy level today?

How were your moods today?

How many hours did you sleep last night?

What step (if any) do you need to focus on tomorrow?

Daily Food Diary

Hunger Scale:

10   Thanksgiving stuffed--You ate too much and are slightly uncomfortable

5   Comfortable

3   You're a little bit hungry, but you could wait

0   Your stomach is empty

Try to eat in the range of 0 to 5 for best results

TIME	FOOD	Hunger # before eating	Hunger # after eating

THE DAILY CHECKLIST

Day & Date _____

☐ 1. Keep track of what you're eating

☐ 2. Eat breakfast within an hour of waking up.

☐ 3. Wait until you are hungry to eat (except for rule #2).

☐ 4. Eat protein & carb at every meal/snack.

☐ 5. Eat a vegetable or fruit every time you eat.

Fruit ☐ ☐ | Vegetables ☐ ☐ ☐

☐ 6. Eat 25 g of fiber each day. Today approx. total: _____ g

☐ 7. Drink 8-10 glasses of water daily. ☐ ☐ ☐ ☐ ☐ ☐ ☐ ☐ ☐

☐ 8. Stop eating 2 hours before bedtime.

☐ 9. No junk food & limited alcohol.

☐ 10. Stop eating when satisfied, not full.

How many steps did you follow today? ___/10

What was your "grade" today? __ (A or B is your goal)

9 or 10/10 = A
8 of 10 = B
7 of 10 = C
Less than that? Just strive for better tomorrow, okay? No big deal. Remember, you're always just one meal or snack away from being back on your plan.

How was your energy level today?

How were your moods today?

How many hours did you sleep last night?

What step (if any) do you need to focus on tomorrow?

Daily Food Diary

Hunger Scale:

10   Thanksgiving stuffed--You ate too much and are slightly uncomfortable

5   Comfortable

3   You're a little bit hungry, but you could wait

0   Your stomach is empty

Try to eat in the range of 0 to 5 for best results

TIME	FOOD	Hunger # before eating	Hunger # after eating

THE DAILY CHECKLIST

Day & Date _____

☐ 1. Keep track of what you're eating

☐ 2. Eat breakfast within an hour of waking up.

☐ 3. Wait until you are hungry to eat (except for rule #2).

☐ 4. Eat protein & carb at every meal/snack.

☐ 5. Eat a vegetable or fruit every time you eat.

    Fruit ☐ ☐ | Vegetables ☐ ☐ ☐

☐ 6. Eat 25 g of fiber each day. Today approx. total: _____ g

☐ 7. Drink 8-10 glasses of water daily. ☐ ☐ ☐ ☐ ☐ ☐ ☐ ☐ ☐

☐ 8. Stop eating 2 hours before bedtime.

☐ 9. No junk food & limited alcohol.

☐ 10. Stop eating when satisfied, not full.

How many steps did you follow today? ___/10

What was your "grade" today? __ (A or B is your goal)

9 or 10/10 = A
8 of 10 = B
7 of 10 = C
Less than that? Just strive for better tomorrow, okay? No big deal. Remember, you're always just one meal or snack away from being back on your plan.

How was your energy level today?

How were your moods today?

How many hours did you sleep last night?

What step (if any) do you need to focus on tomorrow?

Daily Food Diary

Hunger Scale:

10   Thanksgiving stuffed--You ate too much and are slightly uncomfortable

5   Comfortable

3   You're a little bit hungry, but you could wait

0   Your stomach is empty

Try to eat in the range of 0 to 5 for best results

TIME	FOOD	Hunger # before eating	Hunger # after eating

Rebecca J. Clark

PERIODIC CHECK-IN

What is your weight today?

If you're trying to lose weight, did you? And if so, how much?

How have you been doing on your Checklist? Has it been easy/hard?

Are there any steps you're consistently skipping? If so, which one(s)?

If there is a step or more that you've been skipping, strive to focus on it starting now.

Nice job! You're doing great.

NOTES:

THE DAILY CHECKLIST
Day & Date _____

☐ 1. Keep track of what you're eating

☐ 2. Eat breakfast within an hour of waking up.

☐ 3. Wait until you are hungry to eat (except for rule #2).

☐ 4. Eat protein & carb at every meal/snack.

☐ 5. Eat a vegetable or fruit every time you eat.

  Fruit ☐ ☐ | Vegetables ☐ ☐ ☐

☐ 6. Eat 25 g of fiber each day. Today approx. total: _____ g

☐ 7. Drink 8-10 glasses of water daily. ☐ ☐ ☐ ☐ ☐ ☐ ☐ ☐ ☐

☐ 8. Stop eating 2 hours before bedtime.

☐ 9. No junk food & limited alcohol.

☐ 10. Stop eating when satisfied, not full.

How many steps did you follow today? ___/10

What was your "grade" today? __ (A or B is your goal)

9 or 10/10 = A
8 of 10 = B
7 of 10 = C
Less than that? Just strive for better tomorrow, okay? No big deal. Remember, you're always just one meal or snack away from being back on your plan.

How was your energy level today?

How were your moods today?

How many hours did you sleep last night?

What step (if any) do you need to focus on tomorrow?

Daily Food Diary

Hunger Scale:

10   Thanksgiving stuffed--You ate too much and are slightly uncomfortable

5   Comfortable

3   You're a little bit hungry, but you could wait

0   Your stomach is empty

Try to eat in the range of 0 to 5 for best results

TIME	FOOD	Hunger # before eating	Hunger # after eating

THE DAILY CHECKLIST

Day & Date _____

☐ 1. Keep track of what you're eating

☐ 2. Eat breakfast within an hour of waking up.

☐ 3. Wait until you are hungry to eat (except for rule #2).

☐ 4. Eat protein & carb at every meal/snack.

☐ 5. Eat a vegetable or fruit every time you eat.

  Fruit ☐ ☐ | Vegetables ☐ ☐ ☐

☐ 6. Eat 25 g of fiber each day. Today approx. total: _____ g

☐ 7. Drink 8-10 glasses of water daily. ☐ ☐ ☐ ☐ ☐ ☐ ☐ ☐ ☐

☐ 8. Stop eating 2 hours before bedtime.

☐ 9. No junk food & limited alcohol.

☐ 10. Stop eating when satisfied, not full.

How many steps did you follow today? __/10

What was your "grade" today? __ (A or B is your goal)

9 or 10/10 = A
8 of 10 = B
7 of 10 = C
Less than that? Just strive for better tomorrow, okay? No big deal. Remember, you're always just one meal or snack away from being back on your plan.

How was your energy level today?

How were your moods today?

How many hours did you sleep last night?

What step (if any) do you need to focus on tomorrow?

Daily Food Diary

Hunger Scale:

10   Thanksgiving stuffed--You ate too much and are slightly uncomfortable

5   Comfortable

3   You're a little bit hungry, but you could wait

0   Your stomach is empty

Try to eat in the range of 0 to 5 for best results

TIME	FOOD	Hunger # before eating	Hunger # after eating

THE DAILY CHECKLIST

Day & Date _____

☐ 1. Keep track of what you're eating

☐ 2. Eat breakfast within an hour of waking up.

☐ 3. Wait until you are hungry to eat (except for rule #2).

☐ 4. Eat protein & carb at every meal/snack.

☐ 5. Eat a vegetable or fruit every time you eat.

Fruit ☐ ☐ | Vegetables ☐ ☐ ☐

☐ 6. Eat 25 g of fiber each day. Today approx. total: _____ g

☐ 7. Drink 8-10 glasses of water daily. ☐ ☐ ☐ ☐ ☐ ☐ ☐ ☐ ☐

☐ 8. Stop eating 2 hours before bedtime.

☐ 9. No junk food & limited alcohol.

☐ 10. Stop eating when satisfied, not full.

How many steps did you follow today? ___/10

What was your "grade" today? __ (A or B is your goal)

9 or 10/10 = A
8 of 10 = B
7 of 10 = C
Less than that? Just strive for better tomorrow, okay? No big deal. Remember, you're always just one meal or snack away from being back on your plan.

How was your energy level today?

How were your moods today?

How many hours did you sleep last night?

What step (if any) do you need to focus on tomorrow?

Daily Food Diary

Hunger Scale:

10   Thanksgiving stuffed--You ate too much and are slightly uncomfortable

5   Comfortable

3   You're a little bit hungry, but you could wait

0   Your stomach is empty

Try to eat in the range of 0 to 5 for best results

TIME	FOOD	Hunger # before eating	Hunger # after eating

THE DAILY CHECKLIST

Day & Date _____

☐ 1. Keep track of what you're eating

☐ 2. Eat breakfast within an hour of waking up.

☐ 3. Wait until you are hungry to eat (except for rule #2).

☐ 4. Eat protein & carb at every meal/snack.

☐ 5. Eat a vegetable or fruit every time you eat.

   Fruit ☐ ☐ | Vegetables ☐ ☐ ☐

☐ 6. Eat 25 g of fiber each day. Today approx. total: _____ g

☐ 7. Drink 8-10 glasses of water daily. ☐ ☐ ☐ ☐ ☐ ☐ ☐ ☐ ☐

☐ 8. Stop eating 2 hours before bedtime.

☐ 9. No junk food & limited alcohol.

☐ 10. Stop eating when satisfied, not full.

How many steps did you follow today? ___/10

What was your "grade" today? __ (A or B is your goal)

9 or 10/10 = A
8 of 10 = B
7 of 10 = C
Less than that? Just strive for better tomorrow, okay? No big deal.
Remember, you're always just one meal or snack away from being
back on your plan.

How was your energy level today?

How were your moods today?

How many hours did you sleep last night?

What step (if any) do you need to focus on tomorrow?

Daily Food Diary

Hunger Scale:

10   Thanksgiving stuffed--You ate too much and are slightly uncomfortable

5   Comfortable

3   You're a little bit hungry, but you could wait

0   Your stomach is empty

Try to eat in the range of 0 to 5 for best results

TIME	FOOD	Hunger # before eating	Hunger # after eating

THE DAILY CHECKLIST

Day & Date _____

☐ 1. Keep track of what you're eating

☐ 2. Eat breakfast within an hour of waking up.

☐ 3. Wait until you are hungry to eat (except for rule #2).

☐ 4. Eat protein & carb at every meal/snack.

☐ 5. Eat a vegetable or fruit every time you eat.

    Fruit ☐ ☐ | Vegetables ☐ ☐ ☐

☐ 6. Eat 25 g of fiber each day. Today approx. total: _____ g

☐ 7. Drink 8-10 glasses of water daily. ☐ ☐ ☐ ☐ ☐ ☐ ☐ ☐ ☐

☐ 8. Stop eating 2 hours before bedtime.

☐ 9. No junk food & limited alcohol.

☐ 10. Stop eating when satisfied, not full.

How many steps did you follow today? ___/10

What was your "grade" today? __ (A or B is your goal)

9 or 10/10 = A
8 of 10 = B
7 of 10 = C
Less than that? Just strive for better tomorrow, okay? No big deal. Remember, you're always just one meal or snack away from being back on your plan.

How was your energy level today?

How were your moods today?

How many hours did you sleep last night?

What step (if any) do you need to focus on tomorrow?

Daily Food Diary

Hunger Scale:

10   Thanksgiving stuffed--You ate too much and are slightly uncomfortable

5   Comfortable

3   You're a little bit hungry, but you could wait

0   Your stomach is empty

Try to eat in the range of 0 to 5 for best results

TIME	FOOD	Hunger # before eating	Hunger # after eating

THE DAILY CHECKLIST

Day & Date _____

☐ 1. Keep track of what you're eating

☐ 2. Eat breakfast within an hour of waking up.

☐ 3. Wait until you are hungry to eat (except for rule #2).

☐ 4. Eat protein & carb at every meal/snack.

☐ 5. Eat a vegetable or fruit every time you eat.

    Fruit ☐ ☐ | Vegetables ☐ ☐ ☐

☐ 6. Eat 25 g of fiber each day. Today approx. total: _____ g

☐ 7. Drink 8-10 glasses of water daily. ☐ ☐ ☐ ☐ ☐ ☐ ☐ ☐ ☐

☐ 8. Stop eating 2 hours before bedtime.

☐ 9. No junk food & limited alcohol.

☐ 10. Stop eating when satisfied, not full.

How many steps did you follow today? __/10

What was your "grade" today? _ (A or B is your goal)

9 or 10/10 = A
8 of 10 = B
7 of 10 = C
Less than that? Just strive for better tomorrow, okay? No big deal. Remember, you're always just one meal or snack away from being back on your plan.

How was your energy level today?

How were your moods today?

How many hours did you sleep last night?

What step (if any) do you need to focus on tomorrow?

Daily Food Diary

Hunger Scale:

10   Thanksgiving stuffed--You ate too much and are slightly uncomfortable

5   Comfortable

3   You're a little bit hungry, but you could wait

0   Your stomach is empty

Try to eat in the range of 0 to 5 for best results

TIME	FOOD	Hunger # before eating	Hunger # after eating

THE DAILY CHECKLIST

Day & Date _____

☐ 1. Keep track of what you're eating

☐ 2. Eat breakfast within an hour of waking up.

☐ 3. Wait until you are hungry to eat (except for rule #2).

☐ 4. Eat protein & carb at every meal/snack.

☐ 5. Eat a vegetable or fruit every time you eat.

      Fruit ☐ ☐ | Vegetables ☐ ☐ ☐

☐ 6. Eat 25 g of fiber each day. Today approx. total: _____ g

☐ 7. Drink 8-10 glasses of water daily. ☐ ☐ ☐ ☐ ☐ ☐ ☐ ☐ ☐

☐ 8. Stop eating 2 hours before bedtime.

☐ 9. No junk food & limited alcohol.

☐ 10. Stop eating when satisfied, not full.

How many steps did you follow today? ___/10

What was your "grade" today? __ (A or B is your goal)

9 or 10/10 = A
8 of 10 = B
7 of 10 = C
Less than that? Just strive for better tomorrow, okay? No big deal. Remember, you're always just one meal or snack away from being back on your plan.

How was your energy level today?

How were your moods today?

How many hours did you sleep last night?

What step (if any) do you need to focus on tomorrow?

Daily Food Diary

Hunger Scale:

10   Thanksgiving stuffed--You ate too much and are slightly uncomfortable

5   Comfortable

3   You're a little bit hungry, but you could wait

0   Your stomach is empty

Try to eat in the range of 0 to 5 for best results

TIME	FOOD	Hunger # before eating	Hunger # after eating

THE DAILY CHECKLIST

Day & Date _____

☐ 1. Keep track of what you're eating

☐ 2. Eat breakfast within an hour of waking up.

☐ 3. Wait until you are hungry to eat (except for rule #2).

☐ 4. Eat protein & carb at every meal/snack.

☐ 5. Eat a vegetable or fruit every time you eat.

    Fruit ☐ ☐ | Vegetables ☐ ☐ ☐

☐ 6. Eat 25 g of fiber each day. Today approx. total: _____ g

☐ 7. Drink 8-10 glasses of water daily. ☐ ☐ ☐ ☐ ☐ ☐ ☐ ☐

☐ 8. Stop eating 2 hours before bedtime.

☐ 9. No junk food & limited alcohol.

☐ 10. Stop eating when satisfied, not full.

How many steps did you follow today? ___/10

What was your "grade" today? __ (A or B is your goal)

9 or 10/10 = A
8 of 10 = B
7 of 10 = C
Less than that? Just strive for better tomorrow, okay? No big deal.
Remember, you're always just one meal or snack away from being
back on your plan.

How was your energy level today?

How were your moods today?

How many hours did you sleep last night?

What step (if any) do you need to focus on tomorrow?

Daily Food Diary

Hunger Scale:

10   Thanksgiving stuffed--You ate too much and are slightly uncomfortable

5   Comfortable

3   You're a little bit hungry, but you could wait

0   Your stomach is empty

Try to eat in the range of 0 to 5 for best results

TIME	FOOD	Hunger # before eating	Hunger # after eating

THE DAILY CHECKLIST

Day & Date _____

☐ 1. Keep track of what you're eating

☐ 2. Eat breakfast within an hour of waking up.

☐ 3. Wait until you are hungry to eat (except for rule #2).

☐ 4. Eat protein & carb at every meal/snack.

☐ 5. Eat a vegetable or fruit every time you eat.

   Fruit ☐ ☐ | Vegetables ☐ ☐ ☐

☐ 6. Eat 25 g of fiber each day. Today approx. total: _____ g

☐ 7. Drink 8-10 glasses of water daily. ☐ ☐ ☐ ☐ ☐ ☐ ☐ ☐ ☐

☐ 8. Stop eating 2 hours before bedtime.

☐ 9. No junk food & limited alcohol.

☐ 10. Stop eating when satisfied, not full.

How many steps did you follow today? ___/10

What was your "grade" today? __ (A or B is your goal)

9 or 10/10 = A
8 of 10 = B
7 of 10 = C
Less than that? Just strive for better tomorrow, okay? No big deal. Remember, you're always just one meal or snack away from being back on your plan.

How was your energy level today?

How were your moods today?

How many hours did you sleep last night?

What step (if any) do you need to focus on tomorrow?

Daily Food Diary

Hunger Scale:

10   Thanksgiving stuffed--You ate too much and are slightly uncomfortable

5   Comfortable

3   You're a little bit hungry, but you could wait

0   Your stomach is empty

Try to eat in the range of 0 to 5 for best results

TIME	FOOD	Hunger # before eating	Hunger # after eating

THE DAILY CHECKLIST

Day & Date _____

☐ 1. Keep track of what you're eating

☐ 2. Eat breakfast within an hour of waking up.

☐ 3. Wait until you are hungry to eat (except for rule #2).

☐ 4. Eat protein & carb at every meal/snack.

☐ 5. Eat a vegetable or fruit every time you eat.

   Fruit ☐ ☐ | Vegetables ☐ ☐ ☐

☐ 6. Eat 25 g of fiber each day. Today approx. total: _____ g

☐ 7. Drink 8-10 glasses of water daily. ☐ ☐ ☐ ☐ ☐ ☐ ☐ ☐ ☐

☐ 8. Stop eating 2 hours before bedtime.

☐ 9. No junk food & limited alcohol.

☐ 10. Stop eating when satisfied, not full.

How many steps did you follow today? ___/10

What was your "grade" today? __ (A or B is your goal)

9 or 10/10 = A
8 of 10 = B
7 of 10 = C
Less than that? Just strive for better tomorrow, okay? No big deal.
Remember, you're always just one meal or snack away from being
back on your plan.

How was your energy level today?

How were your moods today?

How many hours did you sleep last night?

What step (if any) do you need to focus on tomorrow?

Daily Food Diary

Hunger Scale:

10   Thanksgiving stuffed--You ate too much and are slightly uncomfortable

5   Comfortable

3   You're a little bit hungry, but you could wait

0   Your stomach is empty

Try to eat in the range of 0 to 5 for best results

TIME	FOOD	Hunger # before eating	Hunger # after eating

Rebecca J. Clark

PERIODIC CHECK-IN

What is your weight today?

If you're trying to lose weight, did you? And if so, how much?

How have you been doing on your Checklist? Has it been easy/hard?

Are there any steps you're consistently skipping? If so, which one(s)?

If there is a step or more that you've been skipping, strive to focus on it starting now.

Nice job! You're doing great.

NOTES:

THE DAILY CHECKLIST

Day & Date _____

☐ 1. Keep track of what you're eating

☐ 2. Eat breakfast within an hour of waking up.

☐ 3. Wait until you are hungry to eat (except for rule #2).

☐ 4. Eat protein & carb at every meal/snack.

☐ 5. Eat a vegetable or fruit every time you eat.

   Fruit ☐ ☐ | Vegetables ☐ ☐ ☐

☐ 6. Eat 25 g of fiber each day. Today approx. total: _____ g

☐ 7. Drink 8-10 glasses of water daily. ☐ ☐ ☐ ☐ ☐ ☐ ☐ ☐ ☐

☐ 8. Stop eating 2 hours before bedtime.

☐ 9. No junk food & limited alcohol.

☐ 10. Stop eating when satisfied, not full.

How many steps did you follow today? ___/10

What was your "grade" today? __ (A or B is your goal)

9 or 10/10 = A
8 of 10 = B
7 of 10 = C
Less than that? Just strive for better tomorrow, okay? No big deal. Remember, you're always just one meal or snack away from being back on your plan.

How was your energy level today?

How were your moods today?

How many hours did you sleep last night?

What step (if any) do you need to focus on tomorrow?

Daily Food Diary

Hunger Scale:

10   Thanksgiving stuffed--You ate too much and are slightly uncomfortable

5   Comfortable

3   You're a little bit hungry, but you could wait

0   Your stomach is empty

Try to eat in the range of 0 to 5 for best results

TIME	FOOD	Hunger # before eating	Hunger # after eating

THE DAILY CHECKLIST

Day & Date _____

☐ 1. Keep track of what you're eating

☐ 2. Eat breakfast within an hour of waking up.

☐ 3. Wait until you are hungry to eat (except for rule #2).

☐ 4. Eat protein & carb at every meal/snack.

☐ 5. Eat a vegetable or fruit every time you eat.

     Fruit ☐ ☐ | Vegetables ☐ ☐ ☐

☐ 6. Eat 25 g of fiber each day. Today approx. total: _____ g

☐ 7. Drink 8-10 glasses of water daily. ☐ ☐ ☐ ☐ ☐ ☐ ☐ ☐ ☐

☐ 8. Stop eating 2 hours before bedtime.

☐ 9. No junk food & limited alcohol.

☐ 10. Stop eating when satisfied, not full.

How many steps did you follow today? ___/10

What was your "grade" today? __ (A or B is your goal)

9 or 10/10 = A
8 of 10 = B
7 of 10 = C
Less than that? Just strive for better tomorrow, okay? No big deal.
Remember, you're always just one meal or snack away from being
back on your plan.

How was your energy level today?

How were your moods today?

How many hours did you sleep last night?

What step (if any) do you need to focus on tomorrow?

Daily Food Diary

Hunger Scale:

10   Thanksgiving stuffed--You ate too much and are slightly uncomfortable

5   Comfortable

3   You're a little bit hungry, but you could wait

0   Your stomach is empty

Try to eat in the range of 0 to 5 for best results

TIME	FOOD	Hunger # before eating	Hunger # after eating

THE DAILY CHECKLIST

Day & Date _____

☐ 1. Keep track of what you're eating

☐ 2. Eat breakfast within an hour of waking up.

☐ 3. Wait until you are hungry to eat (except for rule #2).

☐ 4. Eat protein & carb at every meal/snack.

☐ 5. Eat a vegetable or fruit every time you eat.

   Fruit ☐ ☐ | Vegetables ☐ ☐ ☐

☐ 6. Eat 25 g of fiber each day. Today approx. total: _____ g

☐ 7. Drink 8-10 glasses of water daily. ☐ ☐ ☐ ☐ ☐ ☐ ☐ ☐ ☐

☐ 8. Stop eating 2 hours before bedtime.

☐ 9. No junk food & limited alcohol.

☐ 10. Stop eating when satisfied, not full.

How many steps did you follow today? ___/10

What was your "grade" today? __ (A or B is your goal)

9 or 10/10 = A
8 of 10 = B
7 of 10 = C
Less than that? Just strive for better tomorrow, okay? No big deal. Remember, you're always just one meal or snack away from being back on your plan.

How was your energy level today?

How were your moods today?

How many hours did you sleep last night?

What step (if any) do you need to focus on tomorrow?

Daily Food Diary

Hunger Scale:

10   Thanksgiving stuffed--You ate too much and are slightly uncomfortable

5   Comfortable

3   You're a little bit hungry, but you could wait

0   Your stomach is empty

Try to eat in the range of 0 to 5 for best results

TIME	FOOD	Hunger # before eating	Hunger # after eating

THE DAILY CHECKLIST

Day & Date _____

☐ 1. Keep track of what you're eating

☐ 2. Eat breakfast within an hour of waking up.

☐ 3. Wait until you are hungry to eat (except for rule #2).

☐ 4. Eat protein & carb at every meal/snack.

☐ 5. Eat a vegetable or fruit every time you eat.

　　Fruit ☐ ☐ | Vegetables ☐ ☐ ☐

☐ 6. Eat 25 g of fiber each day. Today approx. total: _____ g

☐ 7. Drink 8-10 glasses of water daily. ☐ ☐ ☐ ☐ ☐ ☐ ☐ ☐ ☐

☐ 8. Stop eating 2 hours before bedtime.

☐ 9. No junk food & limited alcohol.

☐ 10. Stop eating when satisfied, not full.

How many steps did you follow today? ___/10

What was your "grade" today? __ (A or B is your goal)

9 or 10/10 = A
8 of 10 = B
7 of 10 = C
Less than that? Just strive for better tomorrow, okay? No big deal. Remember, you're always just one meal or snack away from being back on your plan.

How was your energy level today?

How were your moods today?

How many hours did you sleep last night?

What step (if any) do you need to focus on tomorrow?

Daily Food Diary

Hunger Scale:

10   Thanksgiving stuffed--You ate too much and are slightly uncomfortable

5   Comfortable

3   You're a little bit hungry, but you could wait

0   Your stomach is empty

Try to eat in the range of 0 to 5 for best results

TIME	FOOD	Hunger # before eating	Hunger # after eating

THE DAILY CHECKLIST

Day & Date _____

☐ 1. Keep track of what you're eating

☐ 2. Eat breakfast within an hour of waking up.

☐ 3. Wait until you are hungry to eat (except for rule #2).

☐ 4. Eat protein & carb at every meal/snack.

☐ 5. Eat a vegetable or fruit every time you eat.

      Fruit ☐ ☐ | Vegetables ☐ ☐ ☐

☐ 6. Eat 25 g of fiber each day. Today approx. total: _____ g

☐ 7. Drink 8-10 glasses of water daily. ☐ ☐ ☐ ☐ ☐ ☐ ☐ ☐ ☐

☐ 8. Stop eating 2 hours before bedtime.

☐ 9. No junk food & limited alcohol.

☐ 10. Stop eating when satisfied, not full.

How many steps did you follow today? ___/10

What was your "grade" today? __ (A or B is your goal)

9 or 10/10 = A
8 of 10 = B
7 of 10 = C
Less than that? Just strive for better tomorrow, okay? No big deal.
Remember, you're always just one meal or snack away from being
back on your plan.

How was your energy level today?

How were your moods today?

How many hours did you sleep last night?

What step (if any) do you need to focus on tomorrow?

Daily Food Diary

Hunger Scale:

10   Thanksgiving stuffed--You ate too much and are slightly uncomfortable

5   Comfortable

3   You're a little bit hungry, but you could wait

0   Your stomach is empty

Try to eat in the range of 0 to 5 for best results

TIME	FOOD	Hunger # before eating	Hunger # after eating

THE DAILY CHECKLIST

Day & Date _____

☐ 1. Keep track of what you're eating

☐ 2. Eat breakfast within an hour of waking up.

☐ 3. Wait until you are hungry to eat (except for rule #2).

☐ 4. Eat protein & carb at every meal/snack.

☐ 5. Eat a vegetable or fruit every time you eat.

　　　Fruit ☐ ☐ | Vegetables ☐ ☐ ☐

☐ 6. Eat 25 g of fiber each day. Today approx. total: _____ g

☐ 7. Drink 8-10 glasses of water daily. ☐ ☐ ☐ ☐ ☐ ☐ ☐ ☐ ☐

☐ 8. Stop eating 2 hours before bedtime.

☐ 9. No junk food & limited alcohol.

☐ 10. Stop eating when satisfied, not full.

How many steps did you follow today? ___/10

What was your "grade" today? __ (A or B is your goal)

9 or 10/10 = A
8 of 10 = B
7 of 10 = C
Less than that? Just strive for better tomorrow, okay? No big deal. Remember, you're always just one meal or snack away from being back on your plan.

How was your energy level today?

How were your moods today?

How many hours did you sleep last night?

What step (if any) do you need to focus on tomorrow?

Daily Food Diary

Hunger Scale:

10   Thanksgiving stuffed--You ate too much and are slightly uncomfortable

5   Comfortable

3   You're a little bit hungry, but you could wait

0   Your stomach is empty

Try to eat in the range of 0 to 5 for best results

TIME	FOOD	Hunger # before eating	Hunger # after eating

Rebecca J. Clark

PERIODIC CHECK-IN

What is your weight today?

If you're trying to lose weight, did you? And if so, how much?

How have you been doing on your Checklist? Has it been easy/hard?

Are there any steps you're consistently skipping? If so, which one(s)?

If there is a step or more that you've been skipping, strive to focus on it starting now.

Nice job! You're doing great.

NOTES:

THE DAILY CHECKLIST

Day & Date _____

☐ 1. Keep track of what you're eating

☐ 2. Eat breakfast within an hour of waking up.

☐ 3. Wait until you are hungry to eat (except for rule #2).

☐ 4. Eat protein & carb at every meal/snack.

☐ 5. Eat a vegetable or fruit every time you eat.

　　Fruit ☐ ☐ | Vegetables ☐ ☐ ☐

☐ 6. Eat 25 g of fiber each day. Today approx. total: _____ g

☐ 7. Drink 8-10 glasses of water daily. ☐ ☐ ☐ ☐ ☐ ☐ ☐ ☐ ☐

☐ 8. Stop eating 2 hours before bedtime.

☐ 9. No junk food & limited alcohol.

☐ 10. Stop eating when satisfied, not full.

How many steps did you follow today? ___/10

What was your "grade" today? __ (A or B is your goal)

9 or 10/10 = A
8 of 10 = B
7 of 10 = C
Less than that? Just strive for better tomorrow, okay? No big deal. Remember, you're always just one meal or snack away from being back on your plan.

How was your energy level today?

How were your moods today?

How many hours did you sleep last night?

What step (if any) do you need to focus on tomorrow?

Daily Food Diary

Hunger Scale:

10 Thanksgiving stuffed--You ate too much and are slightly uncomfortable

5   Comfortable

3   You're a little bit hungry, but you could wait

0   Your stomach is empty

Try to eat in the range of 0 to 5 for best results

TIME	FOOD	Hunger # before eating	Hunger # after eating

THE DAILY CHECKLIST

Day & Date _____

☐ 1. Keep track of what you're eating

☐ 2. Eat breakfast within an hour of waking up.

☐ 3. Wait until you are hungry to eat (except for rule #2).

☐ 4. Eat protein & carb at every meal/snack.

☐ 5. Eat a vegetable or fruit every time you eat.

     Fruit ☐ ☐ | Vegetables ☐ ☐ ☐

☐ 6. Eat 25 g of fiber each day. Today approx. total: _____ g

☐ 7. Drink 8-10 glasses of water daily. ☐ ☐ ☐ ☐ ☐ ☐ ☐ ☐ ☐

☐ 8. Stop eating 2 hours before bedtime.

☐ 9. No junk food & limited alcohol.

☐ 10. Stop eating when satisfied, not full.

How many steps did you follow today? ___/10

What was your "grade" today? __ (A or B is your goal)

9 or 10/10 = A
8 of 10 = B
7 of 10 = C
Less than that? Just strive for better tomorrow, okay? No big deal. Remember, you're always just one meal or snack away from being back on your plan.

How was your energy level today?

How were your moods today?

How many hours did you sleep last night?

What step (if any) do you need to focus on tomorrow?

Daily Food Diary

Hunger Scale:

10   Thanksgiving stuffed--You ate too much and are slightly uncomfortable

5   Comfortable

3   You're a little bit hungry, but you could wait

0   Your stomach is empty

Try to eat in the range of 0 to 5 for best results

TIME	FOOD	Hunger # before eating	Hunger # after eating

THE DAILY CHECKLIST

Day & Date _____

☐ 1. Keep track of what you're eating

☐ 2. Eat breakfast within an hour of waking up.

☐ 3. Wait until you are hungry to eat (except for rule #2).

☐ 4. Eat protein & carb at every meal/snack.

☐ 5. Eat a vegetable or fruit every time you eat.

    Fruit ☐ ☐ | Vegetables ☐ ☐ ☐

☐ 6. Eat 25 g of fiber each day. Today approx. total: _____ g

☐ 7. Drink 8-10 glasses of water daily. ☐ ☐ ☐ ☐ ☐ ☐ ☐ ☐ ☐

☐ 8. Stop eating 2 hours before bedtime.

☐ 9. No junk food & limited alcohol.

☐ 10. Stop eating when satisfied, not full.

How many steps did you follow today? ___/10

What was your "grade" today? __ (A or B is your goal)

9 or 10/10 = A
8 of 10 = B
7 of 10 = C
Less than that? Just strive for better tomorrow, okay? No big deal.
Remember, you're always just one meal or snack away from being
back on your plan.

How was your energy level today?

How were your moods today?

How many hours did you sleep last night?

What step (if any) do you need to focus on tomorrow?

Daily Food Diary

Hunger Scale:

10 Thanksgiving stuffed--You ate too much and are slightly uncomfortable

5 Comfortable

3 You're a little bit hungry, but you could wait

0 Your stomach is empty

Try to eat in the range of 0 to 5 for best results

TIME	FOOD	Hunger # before eating	Hunger # after eating

THE DAILY CHECKLIST

Day & Date _____

☐ 1. Keep track of what you're eating

☐ 2. Eat breakfast within an hour of waking up.

☐ 3. Wait until you are hungry to eat (except for rule #2).

☐ 4. Eat protein & carb at every meal/snack.

☐ 5. Eat a vegetable or fruit every time you eat.

   Fruit ☐ ☐ | Vegetables ☐ ☐ ☐

☐ 6. Eat 25 g of fiber each day. Today approx. total: _____ g

☐ 7. Drink 8-10 glasses of water daily. ☐ ☐ ☐ ☐ ☐ ☐ ☐ ☐ ☐

☐ 8. Stop eating 2 hours before bedtime.

☐ 9. No junk food & limited alcohol.

☐ 10. Stop eating when satisfied, not full.

How many steps did you follow today? ___/10

What was your "grade" today? __ (A or B is your goal)

9 or 10/10 = A
8 of 10 = B
7 of 10 = C
Less than that? Just strive for better tomorrow, okay? No big deal.
Remember, you're always just one meal or snack away from being
back on your plan.

How was your energy level today?

How were your moods today?

How many hours did you sleep last night?

What step (if any) do you need to focus on tomorrow?

Daily Food Diary

Hunger Scale:

10	Thanksgiving stuffed--You ate too much and are slightly uncomfortable
5	Comfortable
3	You're a little bit hungry, but you could wait
0	Your stomach is empty

Try to eat in the range of 0 to 5 for best results

TIME	FOOD	Hunger # before eating	Hunger # after eating

THE DAILY CHECKLIST

Day & Date _____

☐ 1. Keep track of what you're eating

☐ 2. Eat breakfast within an hour of waking up.

☐ 3. Wait until you are hungry to eat (except for rule #2).

☐ 4. Eat protein & carb at every meal/snack.

☐ 5. Eat a vegetable or fruit every time you eat.

    Fruit ☐ ☐ | Vegetables ☐ ☐ ☐

☐ 6. Eat 25 g of fiber each day. Today approx. total: _____ g

☐ 7. Drink 8-10 glasses of water daily. ☐ ☐ ☐ ☐ ☐ ☐ ☐ ☐ ☐

☐ 8. Stop eating 2 hours before bedtime.

☐ 9. No junk food & limited alcohol.

☐ 10. Stop eating when satisfied, not full.

How many steps did you follow today? ___/10

What was your "grade" today? __ (A or B is your goal)

9 or 10/10 = A
8 of 10 = B
7 of 10 = C
Less than that? Just strive for better tomorrow, okay? No big deal. Remember, you're always just one meal or snack away from being back on your plan.

How was your energy level today?

How were your moods today?

How many hours did you sleep last night?

What step (if any) do you need to focus on tomorrow?

The Checklist Diet

Daily Food Diary

Hunger Scale:

10   Thanksgiving stuffed--You ate too much and are slightly uncomfortable

5   Comfortable

3   You're a little bit hungry, but you could wait

0   Your stomach is empty

Try to eat in the range of 0 to 5 for best results

TIME	FOOD	Hunger # before eating	Hunger # after eating

101

THE DAILY CHECKLIST

Day & Date _____

☐ 1. Keep track of what you're eating

☐ 2. Eat breakfast within an hour of waking up.

☐ 3. Wait until you are hungry to eat (except for rule #2).

☐ 4. Eat protein & carb at every meal/snack.

☐ 5. Eat a vegetable or fruit every time you eat.

    Fruit ☐ ☐ | Vegetables ☐ ☐ ☐

☐ 6. Eat 25 g of fiber each day. Today approx. total: _____ g

☐ 7. Drink 8-10 glasses of water daily. ☐ ☐ ☐ ☐ ☐ ☐ ☐ ☐ ☐

☐ 8. Stop eating 2 hours before bedtime.

☐ 9. No junk food & limited alcohol.

☐ 10. Stop eating when satisfied, not full.

How many steps did you follow today? __/10

What was your "grade" today? __ (A or B is your goal)

9 or 10/10 = A
8 of 10 = B
7 of 10 = C
Less than that? Just strive for better tomorrow, okay? No big deal. Remember, you're always just one meal or snack away from being back on your plan.

How was your energy level today?

How were your moods today?

How many hours did you sleep last night?

What step (if any) do you need to focus on tomorrow?

Daily Food Diary

Hunger Scale:

10   Thanksgiving stuffed--You ate too much and are slightly uncomfortable

5   Comfortable

3   You're a little bit hungry, but you could wait

0   Your stomach is empty

Try to eat in the range of 0 to 5 for best results

TIME	FOOD	Hunger # before eating	Hunger # after eating

THE DAILY CHECKLIST
Day & Date _____

☐ 1. Keep track of what you're eating

☐ 2. Eat breakfast within an hour of waking up.

☐ 3. Wait until you are hungry to eat (except for rule #2).

☐ 4. Eat protein & carb at every meal/snack.

☐ 5. Eat a vegetable or fruit every time you eat.

     Fruit ☐ ☐ | Vegetables ☐ ☐ ☐

☐ 6. Eat 25 g of fiber each day. Today approx. total: _____ g

☐ 7. Drink 8-10 glasses of water daily. ☐ ☐ ☐ ☐ ☐ ☐ ☐ ☐ ☐

☐ 8. Stop eating 2 hours before bedtime.

☐ 9. No junk food & limited alcohol.

☐ 10. Stop eating when satisfied, not full.

How many steps did you follow today? ___/10

What was your "grade" today? __ (A or B is your goal)

9 or 10/10 = A
8 of 10 = B
7 of 10 = C
Less than that? Just strive for better tomorrow, okay? No big deal. Remember, you're always just one meal or snack away from being back on your plan.

How was your energy level today?

How were your moods today?

How many hours did you sleep last night?

What step (if any) do you need to focus on tomorrow?

Daily Food Diary

Hunger Scale:

10   Thanksgiving stuffed--You ate too much and are slightly uncomfortable

5   Comfortable

3   You're a little bit hungry, but you could wait

0   Your stomach is empty

Try to eat in the range of 0 to 5 for best results

TIME	FOOD	Hunger # before eating	Hunger # after eating

THE DAILY CHECKLIST

Day & Date _____

☐ 1. Keep track of what you're eating

☐ 2. Eat breakfast within an hour of waking up.

☐ 3. Wait until you are hungry to eat (except for rule #2).

☐ 4. Eat protein & carb at every meal/snack.

☐ 5. Eat a vegetable or fruit every time you eat.

      Fruit ☐ ☐ | Vegetables ☐ ☐ ☐

☐ 6. Eat 25 g of fiber each day. Today approx. total: _____ g

☐ 7. Drink 8-10 glasses of water daily. ☐ ☐ ☐ ☐ ☐ ☐ ☐ ☐ ☐

☐ 8. Stop eating 2 hours before bedtime.

☐ 9. No junk food & limited alcohol.

☐ 10. Stop eating when satisfied, not full.

How many steps did you follow today? ___/10

What was your "grade" today? __ (A or B is your goal)

9 or 10/10 = A
8 of 10 = B
7 of 10 = C
Less than that? Just strive for better tomorrow, okay? No big deal. Remember, you're always just one meal or snack away from being back on your plan.

How was your energy level today?

How were your moods today?

How many hours did you sleep last night?

What step (if any) do you need to focus on tomorrow?

Daily Food Diary

Hunger Scale:

10   Thanksgiving stuffed--You ate too much and are slightly uncomfortable

5   Comfortable

3   You're a little bit hungry, but you could wait

0   Your stomach is empty

Try to eat in the range of 0 to 5 for best results

TIME	FOOD	Hunger # before eating	Hunger # after eating

Rebecca J. Clark

THE DAILY CHECKLIST

Day & Date _____

☐ 1. Keep track of what you're eating

☐ 2. Eat breakfast within an hour of waking up.

☐ 3. Wait until you are hungry to eat (except for rule #2).

☐ 4. Eat protein & carb at every meal/snack.

☐ 5. Eat a vegetable or fruit every time you eat.

    Fruit ☐ ☐ | Vegetables ☐ ☐ ☐

☐ 6. Eat 25 g of fiber each day. Today approx. total: _____ g

☐ 7. Drink 8-10 glasses of water daily. ☐ ☐ ☐ ☐ ☐ ☐ ☐ ☐ ☐

☐ 8. Stop eating 2 hours before bedtime.

☐ 9. No junk food & limited alcohol.

☐ 10. Stop eating when satisfied, not full.

How many steps did you follow today? ___/10

What was your "grade" today? __ (A or B is your goal)

9 or 10/10 = A
8 of 10 = B
7 of 10 = C
Less than that? Just strive for better tomorrow, okay? No big deal. Remember, you're always just one meal or snack away from being back on your plan.

How was your energy level today?

How were your moods today?

How many hours did you sleep last night?

What step (if any) do you need to focus on tomorrow?

Daily Food Diary

Hunger Scale:

10   Thanksgiving stuffed--You ate too much and are slightly uncomfortable

5   Comfortable

3   You're a little bit hungry, but you could wait

0   Your stomach is empty

Try to eat in the range of 0 to 5 for best results

TIME	FOOD	Hunger # before eating	Hunger # after eating

THE DAILY CHECKLIST

Day & Date _____

☐ 1. Keep track of what you're eating

☐ 2. Eat breakfast within an hour of waking up.

☐ 3. Wait until you are hungry to eat (except for rule #2).

☐ 4. Eat protein & carb at every meal/snack.

☐ 5. Eat a vegetable or fruit every time you eat.

    Fruit ☐ ☐ | Vegetables ☐ ☐ ☐

☐ 6. Eat 25 g of fiber each day. Today approx. total: _____ g

☐ 7. Drink 8-10 glasses of water daily. ☐ ☐ ☐ ☐ ☐ ☐ ☐ ☐ ☐

☐ 8. Stop eating 2 hours before bedtime.

☐ 9. No junk food & limited alcohol.

☐ 10. Stop eating when satisfied, not full.

How many steps did you follow today? ___/10

What was your "grade" today? __ (A or B is your goal)

9 or 10/10 = A
8 of 10 = B
7 of 10 = C
Less than that? Just strive for better tomorrow, okay? No big deal. Remember, you're always just one meal or snack away from being back on your plan.

How was your energy level today?

How were your moods today?

How many hours did you sleep last night?

What step (if any) do you need to focus on tomorrow?

Daily Food Diary

Hunger Scale:

10   Thanksgiving stuffed--You ate too much and are slightly uncomfortable

5   Comfortable

3   You're a little bit hungry, but you could wait

0   Your stomach is empty

Try to eat in the range of 0 to 5 for best results

TIME	FOOD	Hunger # before eating	Hunger # after eating

THE DAILY CHECKLIST

Day & Date _____

☐ 1. Keep track of what you're eating

☐ 2. Eat breakfast within an hour of waking up.

☐ 3. Wait until you are hungry to eat (except for rule #2).

☐ 4. Eat protein & carb at every meal/snack.

☐ 5. Eat a vegetable or fruit every time you eat.

      Fruit ☐ ☐ | Vegetables ☐ ☐ ☐

☐ 6. Eat 25 g of fiber each day. Today approx. total: _____ g

☐ 7. Drink 8-10 glasses of water daily. ☐ ☐ ☐ ☐ ☐ ☐ ☐ ☐ ☐

☐ 8. Stop eating 2 hours before bedtime.

☐ 9. No junk food & limited alcohol.

☐ 10. Stop eating when satisfied, not full.

How many steps did you follow today? ___/10

What was your "grade" today? __ (A or B is your goal)

9 or 10/10 = A
8 of 10 = B
7 of 10 = C
Less than that? Just strive for better tomorrow, okay? No big deal.
Remember, you're always just one meal or snack away from being
back on your plan.

How was your energy level today?

How were your moods today?

How many hours did you sleep last night?

What step (if any) do you need to focus on tomorrow?

Daily Food Diary

Hunger Scale:

10	Thanksgiving stuffed--You ate too much and are slightly uncomfortable
5	Comfortable
3	You're a little bit hungry, but you could wait
0	Your stomach is empty

Try to eat in the range of 0 to 5 for best results

TIME	FOOD	Hunger # before eating	Hunger # after eating

PERIODIC CHECK-IN

What is your weight today?

If you're trying to lose weight, did you? And if so, how much?

How have you been doing on your Checklist? Has it been easy/hard?

Are there any steps you're consistently skipping? If so, which one(s)?

If there is a step or more that you've been skipping, strive to focus on it starting now.

Nice job! You're doing great.

NOTES:

THE DAILY CHECKLIST

Day & Date _____

☐ 1. Keep track of what you're eating

☐ 2. Eat breakfast within an hour of waking up.

☐ 3. Wait until you are hungry to eat (except for rule #2).

☐ 4. Eat protein & carb at every meal/snack.

☐ 5. Eat a vegetable or fruit every time you eat.

    Fruit ☐ ☐ | Vegetables ☐ ☐ ☐

☐ 6. Eat 25 g of fiber each day. Today approx. total: _____ g

☐ 7. Drink 8-10 glasses of water daily. ☐ ☐ ☐ ☐ ☐ ☐ ☐ ☐ ☐

☐ 8. Stop eating 2 hours before bedtime.

☐ 9. No junk food & limited alcohol.

☐ 10. Stop eating when satisfied, not full.

How many steps did you follow today? ___/10

What was your "grade" today? __ (A or B is your goal)

9 or 10/10 = A
8 of 10 = B
7 of 10 = C
Less than that? Just strive for better tomorrow, okay? No big deal.
Remember, you're always just one meal or snack away from being
back on your plan.

How was your energy level today?

How were your moods today?

How many hours did you sleep last night?

What step (if any) do you need to focus on tomorrow?

Daily Food Diary

Hunger Scale:

10   Thanksgiving stuffed--You ate too much and are slightly uncomfortable

5   Comfortable

3   You're a little bit hungry, but you could wait

0   Your stomach is empty

Try to eat in the range of 0 to 5 for best results

TIME	FOOD	Hunger # before eating	Hunger # after eating

THE DAILY CHECKLIST

Day & Date _____

☐ 1. Keep track of what you're eating

☐ 2. Eat breakfast within an hour of waking up.

☐ 3. Wait until you are hungry to eat (except for rule #2).

☐ 4. Eat protein & carb at every meal/snack.

☐ 5. Eat a vegetable or fruit every time you eat.

     Fruit ☐ ☐ | Vegetables ☐ ☐ ☐

☐ 6. Eat 25 g of fiber each day. Today approx. total: _____ g

☐ 7. Drink 8-10 glasses of water daily. ☐ ☐ ☐ ☐ ☐ ☐ ☐ ☐ ☐

☐ 8. Stop eating 2 hours before bedtime.

☐ 9. No junk food & limited alcohol.

☐ 10. Stop eating when satisfied, not full.

How many steps did you follow today? __/10

What was your "grade" today? __ (A or B is your goal)

9 or 10/10 = A
8 of 10 = B
7 of 10 = C
Less than that? Just strive for better tomorrow, okay? No big deal. Remember, you're always just one meal or snack away from being back on your plan.

How was your energy level today?

How were your moods today?

How many hours did you sleep last night?

What step (if any) do you need to focus on tomorrow?

Daily Food Diary

Hunger Scale:

10 Thanksgiving stuffed--You ate too much and are slightly uncomfortable

5 Comfortable

3 You're a little bit hungry, but you could wait

0 Your stomach is empty

Try to eat in the range of 0 to 5 for best results

TIME	FOOD	Hunger # before eating	Hunger # after eating

THE DAILY CHECKLIST

Day & Date _____

☐ 1. Keep track of what you're eating

☐ 2. Eat breakfast within an hour of waking up.

☐ 3. Wait until you are hungry to eat (except for rule #2).

☐ 4. Eat protein & carb at every meal/snack.

☐ 5. Eat a vegetable or fruit every time you eat.

     Fruit ☐ ☐ | Vegetables ☐ ☐ ☐

☐ 6. Eat 25 g of fiber each day. Today approx. total: _____ g

☐ 7. Drink 8-10 glasses of water daily. ☐ ☐ ☐ ☐ ☐ ☐ ☐ ☐ ☐

☐ 8. Stop eating 2 hours before bedtime.

☐ 9. No junk food & limited alcohol.

☐ 10. Stop eating when satisfied, not full.

How many steps did you follow today? ___/10

What was your "grade" today? __ (A or B is your goal)

9 or 10/10 = A
8 of 10 = B
7 of 10 = C
Less than that? Just strive for better tomorrow, okay? No big deal.
Remember, you're always just one meal or snack away from being
back on your plan.

How was your energy level today?

How were your moods today?

How many hours did you sleep last night?

What step (if any) do you need to focus on tomorrow?

Daily Food Diary

Hunger Scale:

10 Thanksgiving stuffed--You ate too much and are slightly uncomfortable

5   Comfortable

3   You're a little bit hungry, but you could wait

0   Your stomach is empty

Try to eat in the range of 0 to 5 for best results

TIME	FOOD	Hunger # before eating	Hunger # after eating

THE DAILY CHECKLIST

Day & Date _____

☐ 1. Keep track of what you're eating

☐ 2. Eat breakfast within an hour of waking up.

☐ 3. Wait until you are hungry to eat (except for rule #2).

☐ 4. Eat protein & carb at every meal/snack.

☐ 5. Eat a vegetable or fruit every time you eat.

    Fruit ☐ ☐ | Vegetables ☐ ☐ ☐

☐ 6. Eat 25 g of fiber each day. Today approx. total: _____ g

☐ 7. Drink 8-10 glasses of water daily. ☐ ☐ ☐ ☐ ☐ ☐ ☐ ☐ ☐

☐ 8. Stop eating 2 hours before bedtime.

☐ 9. No junk food & limited alcohol.

☐ 10. Stop eating when satisfied, not full.

How many steps did you follow today? ___/10

What was your "grade" today? __ (A or B is your goal)

9 or 10/10 = A
8 of 10 = B
7 of 10 = C
Less than that? Just strive for better tomorrow, okay? No big deal. Remember, you're always just one meal or snack away from being back on your plan.

How was your energy level today?

How were your moods today?

How many hours did you sleep last night?

What step (if any) do you need to focus on tomorrow?

Daily Food Diary

Hunger Scale:

10 Thanksgiving stuffed--You ate too much and are slightly uncomfortable

5   Comfortable

3   You're a little bit hungry, but you could wait

0   Your stomach is empty

Try to eat in the range of 0 to 5 for best results

TIME	FOOD	Hunger # before eating	Hunger # after eating

THE DAILY CHECKLIST

Day & Date _____

☐ 1. Keep track of what you're eating

☐ 2. Eat breakfast within an hour of waking up.

☐ 3. Wait until you are hungry to eat (except for rule #2).

☐ 4. Eat protein & carb at every meal/snack.

☐ 5. Eat a vegetable or fruit every time you eat.

      Fruit ☐ ☐ | Vegetables ☐ ☐ ☐

☐ 6. Eat 25 g of fiber each day. Today approx. total: _____ g

☐ 7. Drink 8-10 glasses of water daily. ☐ ☐ ☐ ☐ ☐ ☐ ☐ ☐ ☐

☐ 8. Stop eating 2 hours before bedtime.

☐ 9. No junk food & limited alcohol.

☐ 10. Stop eating when satisfied, not full.

How many steps did you follow today? ___/10

What was your "grade" today? __ (A or B is your goal)

9 or 10/10 = A
8 of 10 = B
7 of 10 = C
Less than that? Just strive for better tomorrow, okay? No big deal. Remember, you're always just one meal or snack away from being back on your plan.

How was your energy level today?

How were your moods today?

How many hours did you sleep last night?

What step (if any) do you need to focus on tomorrow?

Daily Food Diary

Hunger Scale:

10 Thanksgiving stuffed--You ate too much and are slightly uncomfortable

5 Comfortable

3 You're a little bit hungry, but you could wait

0 Your stomach is empty

Try to eat in the range of 0 to 5 for best results

TIME	FOOD	Hunger # before eating	Hunger # after eating

THE DAILY CHECKLIST

Day & Date _____

☐ 1. Keep track of what you're eating

☐ 2. Eat breakfast within an hour of waking up.

☐ 3. Wait until you are hungry to eat (except for rule #2).

☐ 4. Eat protein & carb at every meal/snack.

☐ 5. Eat a vegetable or fruit every time you eat.

　　Fruit ☐ ☐ | Vegetables ☐ ☐ ☐

☐ 6. Eat 25 g of fiber each day. Today approx. total: _____ g

☐ 7. Drink 8-10 glasses of water daily. ☐ ☐ ☐ ☐ ☐ ☐ ☐ ☐ ☐

☐ 8. Stop eating 2 hours before bedtime.

☐ 9. No junk food & limited alcohol.

☐ 10. Stop eating when satisfied, not full.

How many steps did you follow today? ___/10

What was your "grade" today? __ (A or B is your goal)

9 or 10/10 = A
8 of 10 = B
7 of 10 = C
Less than that? Just strive for better tomorrow, okay? No big deal. Remember, you're always just one meal or snack away from being back on your plan.

How was your energy level today?

How were your moods today?

How many hours did you sleep last night?

What step (if any) do you need to focus on tomorrow?

Daily Food Diary

Hunger Scale:

10   Thanksgiving stuffed--You ate too much and are slightly uncomfortable

5   Comfortable

3   You're a little bit hungry, but you could wait

0   Your stomach is empty

Try to eat in the range of 0 to 5 for best results

TIME	FOOD	Hunger # before eating	Hunger # after eating

THE DAILY CHECKLIST

Day & Date _____

☐ 1. Keep track of what you're eating

☐ 2. Eat breakfast within an hour of waking up.

☐ 3. Wait until you are hungry to eat (except for rule #2).

☐ 4. Eat protein & carb at every meal/snack.

☐ 5. Eat a vegetable or fruit every time you eat.

      Fruit ☐ ☐ | Vegetables ☐ ☐ ☐

☐ 6. Eat 25 g of fiber each day. Today approx. total: _____ g

☐ 7. Drink 8-10 glasses of water daily. ☐ ☐ ☐ ☐ ☐ ☐ ☐ ☐ ☐

☐ 8. Stop eating 2 hours before bedtime.

☐ 9. No junk food & limited alcohol.

☐ 10. Stop eating when satisfied, not full.

How many steps did you follow today? ___/10

What was your "grade" today? __ (A or B is your goal)

9 or 10/10 = A
8 of 10 = B
7 of 10 = C
Less than that? Just strive for better tomorrow, okay? No big deal. Remember, you're always just one meal or snack away from being back on your plan.

How was your energy level today?

How were your moods today?

How many hours did you sleep last night?

What step (if any) do you need to focus on tomorrow?

Daily Food Diary

Hunger Scale:

10	Thanksgiving stuffed--You ate too much and are slightly uncomfortable
5	Comfortable
3	You're a little bit hungry, but you could wait
0	Your stomach is empty

Try to eat in the range of 0 to 5 for best results

TIME	FOOD	Hunger # before eating	Hunger # after eating

THE DAILY CHECKLIST

Day & Date _____

☐ 1. Keep track of what you're eating

☐ 2. Eat breakfast within an hour of waking up.

☐ 3. Wait until you are hungry to eat (except for rule #2).

☐ 4. Eat protein & carb at every meal/snack.

☐ 5. Eat a vegetable or fruit every time you eat.

      Fruit ☐ ☐ | Vegetables ☐ ☐ ☐

☐ 6. Eat 25 g of fiber each day. Today approx. total: _____ g

☐ 7. Drink 8-10 glasses of water daily. ☐ ☐ ☐ ☐ ☐ ☐ ☐ ☐ ☐

☐ 8. Stop eating 2 hours before bedtime.

☐ 9. No junk food & limited alcohol.

☐ 10. Stop eating when satisfied, not full.

How many steps did you follow today? __/10

What was your "grade" today? _ (A or B is your goal)

9 or 10/10 = A
8 of 10 = B
7 of 10 = C
Less than that? Just strive for better tomorrow, okay? No big deal.
Remember, you're always just one meal or snack away from being
back on your plan.

How was your energy level today?

How were your moods today?

How many hours did you sleep last night?

What step (if any) do you need to focus on tomorrow?

Daily Food Diary

Hunger Scale:

10 Thanksgiving stuffed--You ate too much and are slightly uncomfortable

5   Comfortable

3   You're a little bit hungry, but you could wait

0   Your stomach is empty

Try to eat in the range of 0 to 5 for best results

TIME	FOOD	Hunger # before eating	Hunger # after eating

THE DAILY CHECKLIST

Day & Date _____

☐ 1. Keep track of what you're eating

☐ 2. Eat breakfast within an hour of waking up.

☐ 3. Wait until you are hungry to eat (except for rule #2).

☐ 4. Eat protein & carb at every meal/snack.

☐ 5. Eat a vegetable or fruit every time you eat.

   Fruit ☐ ☐ | Vegetables ☐ ☐ ☐

☐ 6. Eat 25 g of fiber each day. Today approx. total: _____ g

☐ 7. Drink 8-10 glasses of water daily. ☐ ☐ ☐ ☐ ☐ ☐ ☐ ☐ ☐

☐ 8. Stop eating 2 hours before bedtime.

☐ 9. No junk food & limited alcohol.

☐ 10. Stop eating when satisfied, not full.

How many steps did you follow today? ___/10

What was your "grade" today? __ (A or B is your goal)

9 or 10/10 = A
8 of 10 = B
7 of 10 = C
Less than that? Just strive for better tomorrow, okay? No big deal. Remember, you're always just one meal or snack away from being back on your plan.

How was your energy level today?

How were your moods today?

How many hours did you sleep last night?

What step (if any) do you need to focus on tomorrow?

Daily Food Diary

Hunger Scale:

10   Thanksgiving stuffed--You ate too much and are slightly uncomfortable

5   Comfortable

3   You're a little bit hungry, but you could wait

0   Your stomach is empty

Try to eat in the range of 0 to 5 for best results

TIME	FOOD	Hunger # before eating	Hunger # after eating

THE DAILY CHECKLIST
Day & Date _____

- [ ] 1. Keep track of what you're eating
- [ ] 2. Eat breakfast within an hour of waking up.
- [ ] 3. Wait until you are hungry to eat (except for rule #2).
- [ ] 4. Eat protein & carb at every meal/snack.
- [ ] 5. Eat a vegetable or fruit every time you eat.
  - Fruit ☐ ☐ | Vegetables ☐ ☐ ☐
- [ ] 6. Eat 25 g of fiber each day. Today approx. total: _____ g
- [ ] 7. Drink 8-10 glasses of water daily. ☐ ☐ ☐ ☐ ☐ ☐ ☐ ☐ ☐
- [ ] 8. Stop eating 2 hours before bedtime.
- [ ] 9. No junk food & limited alcohol.
- [ ] 10. Stop eating when satisfied, not full.

How many steps did you follow today? ___/10

What was your "grade" today? __ (A or B is your goal)

9 or 10/10 = A
8 of 10 = B
7 of 10 = C
Less than that? Just strive for better tomorrow, okay? No big deal. Remember, you're always just one meal or snack away from being back on your plan.

How was your energy level today?

How were your moods today?

How many hours did you sleep last night?

What step (if any) do you need to focus on tomorrow?

Daily Food Diary

Hunger Scale:

10   Thanksgiving stuffed--You ate too much and are slightly uncomfortable

5   Comfortable

3   You're a little bit hungry, but you could wait

0   Your stomach is empty

Try to eat in the range of 0 to 5 for best results

TIME	FOOD	Hunger # before eating	Hunger # after eating

Rebecca J. Clark

PERIODIC CHECK-IN

What is your weight today?

If you're trying to lose weight, did you? And if so, how much?

How have you been doing on your Checklist? Has it been easy/hard?

Are there any steps you're consistently skipping? If so, which one(s)?

If there is a step or more that you've been skipping,
strive to focus on it starting now.

Nice job! You're doing great.

NOTES:

THE DAILY CHECKLIST

Day & Date _____

☐ 1. Keep track of what you're eating

☐ 2. Eat breakfast within an hour of waking up.

☐ 3. Wait until you are hungry to eat (except for rule #2).

☐ 4. Eat protein & carb at every meal/snack.

☐ 5. Eat a vegetable or fruit every time you eat.

    Fruit ☐ ☐ | Vegetables ☐ ☐ ☐

☐ 6. Eat 25 g of fiber each day. Today approx. total: _____ g

☐ 7. Drink 8-10 glasses of water daily. ☐ ☐ ☐ ☐ ☐ ☐ ☐ ☐ ☐

☐ 8. Stop eating 2 hours before bedtime.

☐ 9. No junk food & limited alcohol.

☐ 10. Stop eating when satisfied, not full.

How many steps did you follow today? ___/10

What was your "grade" today? __ (A or B is your goal)

9 or 10/10 = A
8 of 10 = B
7 of 10 = C
Less than that? Just strive for better tomorrow, okay? No big deal. Remember, you're always just one meal or snack away from being back on your plan.

How was your energy level today?

How were your moods today?

How many hours did you sleep last night?

What step (if any) do you need to focus on tomorrow?

Daily Food Diary

Hunger Scale:

10   Thanksgiving stuffed--You ate too much and are slightly uncomfortable

5   Comfortable

3   You're a little bit hungry, but you could wait

0   Your stomach is empty

Try to eat in the range of 0 to 5 for best results

TIME	FOOD	Hunger # before eating	Hunger # after eating

THE DAILY CHECKLIST

Day & Date _____

☐ 1. Keep track of what you're eating

☐ 2. Eat breakfast within an hour of waking up.

☐ 3. Wait until you are hungry to eat (except for rule #2).

☐ 4. Eat protein & carb at every meal/snack.

☐ 5. Eat a vegetable or fruit every time you eat.

　　Fruit ☐ ☐ | Vegetables ☐ ☐ ☐

☐ 6. Eat 25 g of fiber each day. Today approx. total: _____ g

☐ 7. Drink 8-10 glasses of water daily. ☐ ☐ ☐ ☐ ☐ ☐ ☐ ☐ ☐

☐ 8. Stop eating 2 hours before bedtime.

☐ 9. No junk food & limited alcohol.

☐ 10. Stop eating when satisfied, not full.

How many steps did you follow today? ___/10

What was your "grade" today? __ (A or B is your goal)

9 or 10/10 = A
8 of 10 = B
7 of 10 = C
Less than that? Just strive for better tomorrow, okay? No big deal. Remember, you're always just one meal or snack away from being back on your plan.

How was your energy level today?

How were your moods today?

How many hours did you sleep last night?

What step (if any) do you need to focus on tomorrow?

Daily Food Diary

Hunger Scale:

10   Thanksgiving stuffed--You ate too much and are slightly uncomfortable

5   Comfortable

3   You're a little bit hungry, but you could wait

0   Your stomach is empty

Try to eat in the range of 0 to 5 for best results

TIME	FOOD	Hunger # before eating	Hunger # after eating

THE DAILY CHECKLIST

Day & Date _____

☐ 1. Keep track of what you're eating

☐ 2. Eat breakfast within an hour of waking up.

☐ 3. Wait until you are hungry to eat (except for rule #2).

☐ 4. Eat protein & carb at every meal/snack.

☐ 5. Eat a vegetable or fruit every time you eat.

　　Fruit ☐ ☐ | Vegetables ☐ ☐ ☐

☐ 6. Eat 25 g of fiber each day. Today approx. total: _____ g

☐ 7. Drink 8-10 glasses of water daily. ☐ ☐ ☐ ☐ ☐ ☐ ☐ ☐ ☐

☐ 8. Stop eating 2 hours before bedtime.

☐ 9. No junk food & limited alcohol.

☐ 10. Stop eating when satisfied, not full.

How many steps did you follow today? ___/10

What was your "grade" today? __ (A or B is your goal)

9 or 10/10 = A
8 of 10 = B
7 of 10 = C
Less than that? Just strive for better tomorrow, okay? No big deal. Remember, you're always just one meal or snack away from being back on your plan.

How was your energy level today?

How were your moods today?

How many hours did you sleep last night?

What step (if any) do you need to focus on tomorrow?

Daily Food Diary

Hunger Scale:

10   Thanksgiving stuffed--You ate too much and are slightly uncomfortable

5   Comfortable

3   You're a little bit hungry, but you could wait

0   Your stomach is empty

Try to eat in the range of 0 to 5 for best results

TIME	FOOD	Hunger # before eating	Hunger # after eating

THE DAILY CHECKLIST

Day & Date _____

☐ 1. Keep track of what you're eating

☐ 2. Eat breakfast within an hour of waking up.

☐ 3. Wait until you are hungry to eat (except for rule #2).

☐ 4. Eat protein & carb at every meal/snack.

☐ 5. Eat a vegetable or fruit every time you eat.

    Fruit ☐ ☐ | Vegetables ☐ ☐ ☐

☐ 6. Eat 25 g of fiber each day. Today approx. total: _____ g

☐ 7. Drink 8-10 glasses of water daily. ☐ ☐ ☐ ☐ ☐ ☐ ☐ ☐ ☐

☐ 8. Stop eating 2 hours before bedtime.

☐ 9. No junk food & limited alcohol.

☐ 10. Stop eating when satisfied, not full.

How many steps did you follow today? ___/10

What was your "grade" today? __ (A or B is your goal)

9 or 10/10 = A
8 of 10 = B
7 of 10 = C
Less than that? Just strive for better tomorrow, okay? No big deal. Remember, you're always just one meal or snack away from being back on your plan.

How was your energy level today?

How were your moods today?

How many hours did you sleep last night?

What step (if any) do you need to focus on tomorrow?

Daily Food Diary

Hunger Scale:

10   Thanksgiving stuffed--You ate too much and are slightly uncomfortable

5   Comfortable

3   You're a little bit hungry, but you could wait

0   Your stomach is empty

Try to eat in the range of 0 to 5 for best results

TIME	FOOD	Hunger # before eating	Hunger # after eating

THE DAILY CHECKLIST

Day & Date _____

☐ 1. Keep track of what you're eating

☐ 2. Eat breakfast within an hour of waking up.

☐ 3. Wait until you are hungry to eat (except for rule #2).

☐ 4. Eat protein & carb at every meal/snack.

☐ 5. Eat a vegetable or fruit every time you eat.

　　Fruit ☐ ☐ | Vegetables ☐ ☐ ☐

☐ 6. Eat 25 g of fiber each day. Today approx. total: _____ g

☐ 7. Drink 8-10 glasses of water daily. ☐ ☐ ☐ ☐ ☐ ☐ ☐ ☐ ☐

☐ 8. Stop eating 2 hours before bedtime.

☐ 9. No junk food & limited alcohol.

☐ 10. Stop eating when satisfied, not full.

How many steps did you follow today? __/10

What was your "grade" today? __ (A or B is your goal)

9 or 10/10 = A
8 of 10 = B
7 of 10 = C
Less than that? Just strive for better tomorrow, okay? No big deal. Remember, you're always just one meal or snack away from being back on your plan.

How was your energy level today?

How were your moods today?

How many hours did you sleep last night?

What step (if any) do you need to focus on tomorrow?

Daily Food Diary

Hunger Scale:

10   Thanksgiving stuffed--You ate too much and are slightly uncomfortable

5   Comfortable

3   You're a little bit hungry, but you could wait

0   Your stomach is empty

Try to eat in the range of 0 to 5 for best results

TIME	FOOD	Hunger # before eating	Hunger # after eating

THE DAILY CHECKLIST

Day & Date _____

☐ 1. Keep track of what you're eating

☐ 2. Eat breakfast within an hour of waking up.

☐ 3. Wait until you are hungry to eat (except for rule #2).

☐ 4. Eat protein & carb at every meal/snack.

☐ 5. Eat a vegetable or fruit every time you eat.

   Fruit ☐ ☐ | Vegetables ☐ ☐ ☐

☐ 6. Eat 25 g of fiber each day. Today approx. total: _____ g

☐ 7. Drink 8-10 glasses of water daily. ☐ ☐ ☐ ☐ ☐ ☐ ☐ ☐ ☐

☐ 8. Stop eating 2 hours before bedtime.

☐ 9. No junk food & limited alcohol.

☐ 10. Stop eating when satisfied, not full.

How many steps did you follow today? ___/10

What was your "grade" today? __ (A or B is your goal)

9 or 10/10 = A
8 of 10 = B
7 of 10 = C
Less than that? Just strive for better tomorrow, okay? No big deal. Remember, you're always just one meal or snack away from being back on your plan.

How was your energy level today?

How were your moods today?

How many hours did you sleep last night?

What step (if any) do you need to focus on tomorrow?

Daily Food Diary

Hunger Scale:

10   Thanksgiving stuffed--You ate too much and are slightly uncomfortable

5   Comfortable

3   You're a little bit hungry, but you could wait

0   Your stomach is empty

Try to eat in the range of 0 to 5 for best results

TIME	FOOD	Hunger # before eating	Hunger # after eating

THE DAILY CHECKLIST

Day & Date _____

☐ 1. Keep track of what you're eating

☐ 2. Eat breakfast within an hour of waking up.

☐ 3. Wait until you are hungry to eat (except for rule #2).

☐ 4. Eat protein & carb at every meal/snack.

☐ 5. Eat a vegetable or fruit every time you eat.

     Fruit ☐ ☐ | Vegetables ☐ ☐ ☐

☐ 6. Eat 25 g of fiber each day. Today approx. total: _____ g

☐ 7. Drink 8-10 glasses of water daily. ☐ ☐ ☐ ☐ ☐ ☐ ☐ ☐ ☐

☐ 8. Stop eating 2 hours before bedtime.

☐ 9. No junk food & limited alcohol.

☐ 10. Stop eating when satisfied, not full.

How many steps did you follow today? ___/10

What was your "grade" today? __ (A or B is your goal)

9 or 10/10 = A
8 of 10 = B
7 of 10 = C
Less than that? Just strive for better tomorrow, okay? No big deal. Remember, you're always just one meal or snack away from being back on your plan.

How was your energy level today?

How were your moods today?

How many hours did you sleep last night?

What step (if any) do you need to focus on tomorrow?

Daily Food Diary

Hunger Scale:

10 Thanksgiving stuffed--You ate too much and are slightly uncomfortable

5 Comfortable

3 You're a little bit hungry, but you could wait

0 Your stomach is empty

Try to eat in the range of 0 to 5 for best results

TIME	FOOD	Hunger # before eating	Hunger # after eating

THE DAILY CHECKLIST

Day & Date _____

☐ 1. Keep track of what you're eating

☐ 2. Eat breakfast within an hour of waking up.

☐ 3. Wait until you are hungry to eat (except for rule #2).

☐ 4. Eat protein & carb at every meal/snack.

☐ 5. Eat a vegetable or fruit every time you eat.

    Fruit ☐ ☐ | Vegetables ☐ ☐ ☐

☐ 6. Eat 25 g of fiber each day. Today approx. total: _____ g

☐ 7. Drink 8-10 glasses of water daily. ☐ ☐ ☐ ☐ ☐ ☐ ☐ ☐ ☐

☐ 8. Stop eating 2 hours before bedtime.

☐ 9. No junk food & limited alcohol.

☐ 10. Stop eating when satisfied, not full.

How many steps did you follow today? __/10

What was your "grade" today? __ (A or B is your goal)

9 or 10/10 = A
8 of 10 = B
7 of 10 = C
Less than that? Just strive for better tomorrow, okay? No big deal. Remember, you're always just one meal or snack away from being back on your plan.

How was your energy level today?

How were your moods today?

How many hours did you sleep last night?

What step (if any) do you need to focus on tomorrow?

Daily Food Diary

Hunger Scale:

10   Thanksgiving stuffed--You ate too much and are slightly uncomfortable

5   Comfortable

3   You're a little bit hungry, but you could wait

0   Your stomach is empty

Try to eat in the range of 0 to 5 for best results

TIME	FOOD	Hunger # before eating	Hunger # after eating

THE DAILY CHECKLIST

Day & Date _____

☐ 1. Keep track of what you're eating

☐ 2. Eat breakfast within an hour of waking up.

☐ 3. Wait until you are hungry to eat (except for rule #2).

☐ 4. Eat protein & carb at every meal/snack.

☐ 5. Eat a vegetable or fruit every time you eat.

    Fruit ☐ ☐ | Vegetables ☐ ☐ ☐

☐ 6. Eat 25 g of fiber each day. Today approx. total: _____ g

☐ 7. Drink 8-10 glasses of water daily. ☐ ☐ ☐ ☐ ☐ ☐ ☐ ☐ ☐

☐ 8. Stop eating 2 hours before bedtime.

☐ 9. No junk food & limited alcohol.

☐ 10. Stop eating when satisfied, not full.

How many steps did you follow today? ___/10

What was your "grade" today? __ (A or B is your goal)

9 or 10/10 = A
8 of 10 = B
7 of 10 = C
Less than that? Just strive for better tomorrow, okay? No big deal. Remember, you're always just one meal or snack away from being back on your plan.

How was your energy level today?

How were your moods today?

How many hours did you sleep last night?

What step (if any) do you need to focus on tomorrow?

Daily Food Diary

Hunger Scale:

10   Thanksgiving stuffed--You ate too much and are slightly uncomfortable

5   Comfortable

3   You're a little bit hungry, but you could wait

0   Your stomach is empty

Try to eat in the range of 0 to 5 for best results

TIME	FOOD	Hunger # before eating	Hunger # after eating

THE DAILY CHECKLIST

Day & Date _____

☐ 1. Keep track of what you're eating

☐ 2. Eat breakfast within an hour of waking up.

☐ 3. Wait until you are hungry to eat (except for rule #2).

☐ 4. Eat protein & carb at every meal/snack.

☐ 5. Eat a vegetable or fruit every time you eat.

    Fruit ☐ ☐ | Vegetables ☐ ☐ ☐

☐ 6. Eat 25 g of fiber each day. Today approx. total: _____ g

☐ 7. Drink 8-10 glasses of water daily. ☐ ☐ ☐ ☐ ☐ ☐ ☐ ☐ ☐

☐ 8. Stop eating 2 hours before bedtime.

☐ 9. No junk food & limited alcohol.

☐ 10. Stop eating when satisfied, not full.

How many steps did you follow today? ___/10

What was your "grade" today? __ (A or B is your goal)

9 or 10/10 = A
8 of 10 = B
7 of 10 = C
Less than that? Just strive for better tomorrow, okay? No big deal.
Remember, you're always just one meal or snack away from being
back on your plan.

How was your energy level today?

How were your moods today?

How many hours did you sleep last night?

What step (if any) do you need to focus on tomorrow?

Daily Food Diary

Hunger Scale:

10 Thanksgiving stuffed--You ate too much and are slightly uncomfortable

5   Comfortable

3   You're a little bit hungry, but you could wait

0   Your stomach is empty

Try to eat in the range of 0 to 5 for best results

TIME	FOOD	Hunger # before eating	Hunger # after eating

THE DAILY CHECKLIST

Day & Date _____

☐ 1. Keep track of what you're eating

☐ 2. Eat breakfast within an hour of waking up.

☐ 3. Wait until you are hungry to eat (except for rule #2).

☐ 4. Eat protein & carb at every meal/snack.

☐ 5. Eat a vegetable or fruit every time you eat.

     Fruit ☐ ☐ | Vegetables ☐ ☐ ☐

☐ 6. Eat 25 g of fiber each day. Today approx. total: _____ g

☐ 7. Drink 8-10 glasses of water daily. ☐ ☐ ☐ ☐ ☐ ☐ ☐ ☐ ☐

☐ 8. Stop eating 2 hours before bedtime.

☐ 9. No junk food & limited alcohol.

☐ 10. Stop eating when satisfied, not full.

How many steps did you follow today? ___/10

What was your "grade" today? __ (A or B is your goal)

9 or 10/10 = A
8 of 10 = B
7 of 10 = C
Less than that? Just strive for better tomorrow, okay? No big deal. Remember, you're always just one meal or snack away from being back on your plan.

How was your energy level today?

How were your moods today?

How many hours did you sleep last night?

What step (if any) do you need to focus on tomorrow?

Daily Food Diary

Hunger Scale:

10 Thanksgiving stuffed--You ate too much and are slightly uncomfortable

5 Comfortable

3 You're a little bit hungry, but you could wait

0 Your stomach is empty

Try to eat in the range of 0 to 5 for best results

TIME	FOOD	Hunger # before eating	Hunger # after eating

THE DAILY CHECKLIST

Day & Date _____

☐ 1. Keep track of what you're eating

☐ 2. Eat breakfast within an hour of waking up.

☐ 3. Wait until you are hungry to eat (except for rule #2).

☐ 4. Eat protein & carb at every meal/snack.

☐ 5. Eat a vegetable or fruit every time you eat.

    Fruit ☐ ☐ | Vegetables ☐ ☐ ☐

☐ 6. Eat 25 g of fiber each day. Today approx. total: _____ g

☐ 7. Drink 8-10 glasses of water daily. ☐ ☐ ☐ ☐ ☐ ☐ ☐ ☐ ☐

☐ 8. Stop eating 2 hours before bedtime.

☐ 9. No junk food & limited alcohol.

☐ 10. Stop eating when satisfied, not full.

How many steps did you follow today? ___/10

What was your "grade" today? __ (A or B is your goal)

9 or 10/10 = A
8 of 10 = B
7 of 10 = C
Less than that? Just strive for better tomorrow, okay? No big deal. Remember, you're always just one meal or snack away from being back on your plan.

How was your energy level today?

How were your moods today?

How many hours did you sleep last night?

What step (if any) do you need to focus on tomorrow?

Daily Food Diary

Hunger Scale:

10   Thanksgiving stuffed--You ate too much and are slightly uncomfortable

5   Comfortable

3   You're a little bit hungry, but you could wait

0   Your stomach is empty

Try to eat in the range of 0 to 5 for best results

TIME	FOOD	Hunger # before eating	Hunger # after eating

PERIODIC CHECK-IN

What is your weight today?

If you're trying to lose weight, did you? And if so, how much?

How have you been doing on your Checklist? Has it been easy/hard?

Are there any steps you're consistently skipping? If so, which one(s)?

If there is a step or more that you've been skipping, strive to focus on it starting now.

Nice job! You're doing great.

NOTES:

THE DAILY CHECKLIST

Day & Date _____

☐ 1. Keep track of what you're eating

☐ 2. Eat breakfast within an hour of waking up.

☐ 3. Wait until you are hungry to eat (except for rule #2).

☐ 4. Eat protein & carb at every meal/snack.

☐ 5. Eat a vegetable or fruit every time you eat.

   Fruit ☐ ☐ | Vegetables ☐ ☐ ☐

☐ 6. Eat 25 g of fiber each day. Today approx. total: _____ g

☐ 7. Drink 8-10 glasses of water daily. ☐ ☐ ☐ ☐ ☐ ☐ ☐ ☐ ☐

☐ 8. Stop eating 2 hours before bedtime.

☐ 9. No junk food & limited alcohol.

☐ 10. Stop eating when satisfied, not full.

How many steps did you follow today? ___/10

What was your "grade" today? __ (A or B is your goal)

9 or 10/10 = A
8 of 10 = B
7 of 10 = C
Less than that? Just strive for better tomorrow, okay? No big deal.
Remember, you're always just one meal or snack away from being
back on your plan.

How was your energy level today?

How were your moods today?

How many hours did you sleep last night?

What step (if any) do you need to focus on tomorrow?

Daily Food Diary

Hunger Scale:

10 Thanksgiving stuffed--You ate too much and are slightly uncomfortable

5 Comfortable

3 You're a little bit hungry, but you could wait

0 Your stomach is empty

Try to eat in the range of 0 to 5 for best results

TIME	FOOD	Hunger # before eating	Hunger # after eating

THE DAILY CHECKLIST

Day & Date _____

☐ 1. Keep track of what you're eating

☐ 2. Eat breakfast within an hour of waking up.

☐ 3. Wait until you are hungry to eat (except for rule #2).

☐ 4. Eat protein & carb at every meal/snack.

☐ 5. Eat a vegetable or fruit every time you eat.

      Fruit ☐ ☐ | Vegetables ☐ ☐ ☐

☐ 6. Eat 25 g of fiber each day. Today approx. total: _____ g

☐ 7. Drink 8-10 glasses of water daily. ☐ ☐ ☐ ☐ ☐ ☐ ☐ ☐ ☐

☐ 8. Stop eating 2 hours before bedtime.

☐ 9. No junk food & limited alcohol.

☐ 10. Stop eating when satisfied, not full.

How many steps did you follow today? ___/10

What was your "grade" today? __ (A or B is your goal)

9 or 10/10 = A
8 of 10 = B
7 of 10 = C
Less than that? Just strive for better tomorrow, okay? No big deal.
Remember, you're always just one meal or snack away from being
back on your plan.

How was your energy level today?

How were your moods today?

How many hours did you sleep last night?

What step (if any) do you need to focus on tomorrow?

Daily Food Diary

Hunger Scale:

10   Thanksgiving stuffed--You ate too much and are slightly uncomfortable

5   Comfortable

3   You're a little bit hungry, but you could wait

0   Your stomach is empty

Try to eat in the range of 0 to 5 for best results

TIME	FOOD	Hunger # before eating	Hunger # after eating

THE DAILY CHECKLIST

Day & Date _____

☐ 1. Keep track of what you're eating

☐ 2. Eat breakfast within an hour of waking up.

☐ 3. Wait until you are hungry to eat (except for rule #2).

☐ 4. Eat protein & carb at every meal/snack.

☐ 5. Eat a vegetable or fruit every time you eat.

　　Fruit ☐ ☐ | Vegetables ☐ ☐ ☐

☐ 6. Eat 25 g of fiber each day. Today approx. total: _____ g

☐ 7. Drink 8-10 glasses of water daily. ☐ ☐ ☐ ☐ ☐ ☐ ☐ ☐ ☐

☐ 8. Stop eating 2 hours before bedtime.

☐ 9. No junk food & limited alcohol.

☐ 10. Stop eating when satisfied, not full.

How many steps did you follow today? ___/10

What was your "grade" today? __ (A or B is your goal)

9 or 10/10 = A
8 of 10 = B
7 of 10 = C
Less than that? Just strive for better tomorrow, okay? No big deal. Remember, you're always just one meal or snack away from being back on your plan.

How was your energy level today?

How were your moods today?

How many hours did you sleep last night?

What step (if any) do you need to focus on tomorrow?

Daily Food Diary

Hunger Scale:

10   Thanksgiving stuffed--You ate too much and are slightly uncomfortable

5   Comfortable

3   You're a little bit hungry, but you could wait

0   Your stomach is empty

Try to eat in the range of 0 to 5 for best results

TIME	FOOD	Hunger # before eating	Hunger # after eating

THE DAILY CHECKLIST

Day & Date _____

☐ 1. Keep track of what you're eating

☐ 2. Eat breakfast within an hour of waking up.

☐ 3. Wait until you are hungry to eat (except for rule #2).

☐ 4. Eat protein & carb at every meal/snack.

☐ 5. Eat a vegetable or fruit every time you eat.

    Fruit ☐ ☐ | Vegetables ☐ ☐ ☐

☐ 6. Eat 25 g of fiber each day. Today approx. total: _____ g

☐ 7. Drink 8-10 glasses of water daily. ☐ ☐ ☐ ☐ ☐ ☐ ☐ ☐ ☐

☐ 8. Stop eating 2 hours before bedtime.

☐ 9. No junk food & limited alcohol.

☐ 10. Stop eating when satisfied, not full.

How many steps did you follow today? ___/10

What was your "grade" today? __ (A or B is your goal)

9 or 10/10 = A
8 of 10 = B
7 of 10 = C
Less than that? Just strive for better tomorrow, okay? No big deal. Remember, you're always just one meal or snack away from being back on your plan.

How was your energy level today?

How were your moods today?

How many hours did you sleep last night?

What step (if any) do you need to focus on tomorrow?

Daily Food Diary

Hunger Scale:

10   Thanksgiving stuffed--You ate too much and are slightly uncomfortable

5   Comfortable

3   You're a little bit hungry, but you could wait

0   Your stomach is empty

Try to eat in the range of 0 to 5 for best results

TIME	FOOD	Hunger # before eating	Hunger # after eating

THE DAILY CHECKLIST

Day & Date _____

☐ 1. Keep track of what you're eating

☐ 2. Eat breakfast within an hour of waking up.

☐ 3. Wait until you are hungry to eat (except for rule #2).

☐ 4. Eat protein & carb at every meal/snack.

☐ 5. Eat a vegetable or fruit every time you eat.

    Fruit ☐ ☐ | Vegetables ☐ ☐ ☐

☐ 6. Eat 25 g of fiber each day. Today approx. total: _____ g

☐ 7. Drink 8-10 glasses of water daily. ☐ ☐ ☐ ☐ ☐ ☐ ☐ ☐ ☐

☐ 8. Stop eating 2 hours before bedtime.

☐ 9. No junk food & limited alcohol.

☐ 10. Stop eating when satisfied, not full.

How many steps did you follow today? ___/10

What was your "grade" today? __ (A or B is your goal)

9 or 10/10 = A
8 of 10 = B
7 of 10 = C
Less than that? Just strive for better tomorrow, okay? No big deal.
Remember, you're always just one meal or snack away from being
back on your plan.

How was your energy level today?

How were your moods today?

How many hours did you sleep last night?

What step (if any) do you need to focus on tomorrow?

Daily Food Diary

Hunger Scale:

10   Thanksgiving stuffed--You ate too much and are slightly uncomfortable

5   Comfortable

3   You're a little bit hungry, but you could wait

0   Your stomach is empty

Try to eat in the range of 0 to 5 for best results

TIME	FOOD	Hunger # before eating	Hunger # after eating

THE DAILY CHECKLIST

Day & Date _____

☐ 1. Keep track of what you're eating

☐ 2. Eat breakfast within an hour of waking up.

☐ 3. Wait until you are hungry to eat (except for rule #2).

☐ 4. Eat protein & carb at every meal/snack.

☐ 5. Eat a vegetable or fruit every time you eat.

    Fruit ☐ ☐ | Vegetables ☐ ☐ ☐

☐ 6. Eat 25 g of fiber each day. Today approx. total: _____ g

☐ 7. Drink 8-10 glasses of water daily. ☐ ☐ ☐ ☐ ☐ ☐ ☐ ☐ ☐

☐ 8. Stop eating 2 hours before bedtime.

☐ 9. No junk food & limited alcohol.

☐ 10. Stop eating when satisfied, not full.

How many steps did you follow today? ___/10

What was your "grade" today? __ (A or B is your goal)

9 or 10/10 = A
8 of 10 = B
7 of 10 = C
Less than that? Just strive for better tomorrow, okay? No big deal.
Remember, you're always just one meal or snack away from being
back on your plan.

How was your energy level today?

How were your moods today?

How many hours did you sleep last night?

What step (if any) do you need to focus on tomorrow?

Daily Food Diary

Hunger Scale:

10   Thanksgiving stuffed--You ate too much and are slightly uncomfortable

5   Comfortable

3   You're a little bit hungry, but you could wait

0   Your stomach is empty

Try to eat in the range of 0 to 5 for best results

TIME	FOOD	Hunger # before eating	Hunger # after eating

THE DAILY CHECKLIST

Day & Date _____

☐ 1. Keep track of what you're eating

☐ 2. Eat breakfast within an hour of waking up.

☐ 3. Wait until you are hungry to eat (except for rule #2).

☐ 4. Eat protein & carb at every meal/snack.

☐ 5. Eat a vegetable or fruit every time you eat.

      Fruit ☐ ☐ | Vegetables ☐ ☐ ☐

☐ 6. Eat 25 g of fiber each day. Today approx. total: _____ g

☐ 7. Drink 8-10 glasses of water daily. ☐ ☐ ☐ ☐ ☐ ☐ ☐ ☐ ☐

☐ 8. Stop eating 2 hours before bedtime.

☐ 9. No junk food & limited alcohol.

☐ 10. Stop eating when satisfied, not full.

How many steps did you follow today? ___/10

What was your "grade" today? __ (A or B is your goal)

9 or 10/10 = A
8 of 10 = B
7 of 10 = C
Less than that? Just strive for better tomorrow, okay? No big deal. Remember, you're always just one meal or snack away from being back on your plan.

How was your energy level today?

How were your moods today?

How many hours did you sleep last night?

What step (if any) do you need to focus on tomorrow?

Daily Food Diary

Hunger Scale:

10   Thanksgiving stuffed--You ate too much and are slightly uncomfortable

5   Comfortable

3   You're a little bit hungry, but you could wait

0   Your stomach is empty

Try to eat in the range of 0 to 5 for best results

TIME	FOOD	Hunger # before eating	Hunger # after eating

Rebecca J. Clark

LAST CHECK-IN

So...for the last time... What is your weight today?

If you're trying to lose weight, did you? And if so, how much?

How have you been doing on your Checklist? Has it been easy/hard?

Are there any steps you're consistently skipping? If so, which one(s)?

If there is a step or more that you've been skipping, strive to focus on it starting now.

Nice job! You're doing great.

NOTES:

Food Lists

Use these lists as a guide when choosing what to eat. Is this list exhaustive? Nope. But it'll get you started.

When trying to decide how much to put on your plate, start with a serving size and go from there.

A serving of meat (poultry, beef, pork, fish, etc) is about the size of your palm.
A serving of starchy carbs is about the size of your closed fist.
A serving of fat is about the size of the tip of your thumb.
Unlimited vegetables and fruits (*see Step #5 for details)

HIGH FIBER FOODS (Step #6)
(aim for 25-35 g a day)

Split peas – 16.3 g per cooked cup
Lentils – 15.6 g per cooked cup
Black beans – 15g per cooked cup
Lima beans – 13.2g per cooked cup
Baked beans – 10.4 per cup
Peas – 8.8g per cooked cup
Raspberries – 8 g per cup
Blackberries – 7.6 g per cup
Bran Flakes cereal – 7 g per cup
Avocado – 6.7 g per half avocado
Whole wheat pasta – 6.3 g per cup
Pearl barley – 6 g per cup
Pear – 5.5 g per medium fruit
Broccoli – 5.1g per cooked cup
Oatmeal – 4 g per cooked cup
Corn – 4 g per cooked cup
Brown rice – 3.5 g per cooked cup
Air-popped popcorn – 3.5 g per 3 cups

Almonds – 3.5 g per 1 oz
Banana – 3.1 per medium banana
Strawberries – 3 g per sliced cup

There are many more high-fiber foods, of course, but this list should get you started. When choosing cereal, try to find one that has 5 g of fiber per serving or more. You could also mix your favorite lower fiber cereal with a higher fiber one.

VEGETABLES (Step #5)

Artichokes
Asparagus
Barley
Broccoli
Bok Choy
Cabbage
Carrots
Cauliflower
Celery
Collard Greens
Cucumbers
Eggplant
Lettuce (all varieties)
Mushrooms
Mustard Greens
Okra
Onion
Snow peas
Peppers (all varieties)
Pickles
Radishes
Rhubarb
Sauerkraut
Spinach
Sprouts
Squashes
Tomato
Turnips
Water chestnuts
Zucchini

FRUIT (Step #5)

Apples
Apricots
Blueberries
Cantaloupe
Cherries
Grapefruit
Peaches
Pears

Plums
Strawberries
Raspberries
Blackberries
Nectarines
Watermelon
Bananas
Oranges
Grapes
Pomegranates

PROTEINS (Step #4)

Poultry (prepare these skinless):
Seafood — fish and shellfish
Veal
Ground Beef — extra lean
Beef sirloin
Beef tenderloin
Beef, top round
Lamb
Pork
Canadian bacon
Deli meat — lean choices like chicken, turkey and roast beef
Soy based meat substitutes
Nut Butters
Tofu
Eggs, whole
Eggs, whites
Cheese (limit to 1 oz. per day):
Yogurt (low fat, low sugar only; Greek yogurt has the most protein)
Non-fat or low-fat milk
Soy milk
Almond milk
Cottage cheese
Black Beans
Butter Beans
Chickpeas or Garbanzo Beans
Pinto Beans
Soy Beans
Whey protein powder
Rice protein powder
Soy protein powder
Pea protein powder
Nuts, raw
Lentils
Quinoa (also counts as a carb)

STARCHY CARBS (Step #4)

Bagels — small, whole grain
English muffin — whole grain or sour dough
Bread, multigrain
Bread, rye
Bread, whole wheat
Whole grain cereals
Oatmeal
Pasta, whole wheat or whole grain
Whole grain pita bread
Whole grain flat bread
Popcorn
Potato
Sweet potato
Yam
Rice
Brown rice
Wild rice
Quinoa (also counts as a protein)
Millet

Good luck! I'd love to hear how *The Checklist Diet* works for you. You can contact me with questions or comments, by finding me online.

FIND ME ONLINE
Facebook—authorRebeccaJClark
Twitter @RebeccaJClark
Website – http://RebeccaJClark.com
Newsletter—http://bit.ly/1ebrEDS

Author's note: When I'm not training clients at the awesome little gym where I work, you can find me at home penning romance novels. If you want to know more about my fiction writing, please check out my website (see link above) and/or sign up for my newsletter (which will keep you updated on my fiction *and* nonfiction, plus share healthy tips and recipes).

REBECCA J. CLARK'S FICTION
Borrowed Stilettos
Her One-Night Prince
Deliver the Moon
Shameless
Shameful – prequel to Shameless
Coming soon: Running in Stilettos

www.ingramcontent.com/pod-product-compliance
Lightning Source LLC
Chambersburg PA
CBHW022107280326
41933CB00007B/291